Top Tips
in Urology

EDITED BY

J. McLoughlin MS FRCSUrol
Consultant Urologist,
West Suffolk Hospital,
Bury-St-Edmunds, Suffolk

AND

P.J. O'Boyle ChM FRCS
Consultant Urologist,
Musgrove Park Hospital,
Taunton, Somerset

FOREWORD BY
W.B. Peeling

This publication is provided
as a service to medical education
by ZENECA Pharma

b

**Blackwell
Science**

© 1995 by
Blackwell Science Ltd
Editorial Offices:
Osney Mead, Oxford OX2 0EL
25 John Street, London WC1N 2BL
23 Ainslie Place, Edinburgh EH3 6AJ
238 Main Street, Cambridge
  Massachusetts 02142, USA
54 University Street, Carlton
  Victoria 3053, Australia

Other Editorial Offices:
Arnette Blackwell SA
  1, rue de Lille, 75007 Paris
  France

Blackwell Wissenschafts-Verlag
  GmbH
  Kurfürstendamm 57
  10707 Berlin, Germany

  Feldgasse 13, A-1238 Wien
  Austria

First published 1995

Set by Semantic Graphics, Singapore
Printed and bound in Great Britain
at the Alden Press Limited, Oxford
and Northampton

A catalogue record for this title
is available from the British Library

ISBN 0-86542-610-4

DISTRIBUTORS

  Marston Book Services Ltd
  PO Box 87
  Oxford OX2 0DT
  (*Orders:* Tel: 01865 791155
           Fax: 01865 791927
           Telex: 837515)

North America
  Blackwell Science, Inc.
  238 Main Street
  Cambridge, MA 02142
  (*Orders:* Tel: 800 215-1000
             617 876-7000
           Fax: 617 492-5263)

Australia
  Blackwell Science Pty Ltd
  54 University Street
  Carlton, Victoria 3053
  (*Orders:* Tel: 03 347-0300
           Fax: 03 349-3016)

Library of Congress
Cataloging-in-Publication Data

Top Tips in urology /
edited by J. McLoughlin,
F.J. O'Boyle
        p.   cm.
    Includes bibliographical
    references and index.
    ISBN 0-86542-610-4
    1. Genitourinary organs—
    Surgery—Handbooks, manuals,
    etc.
    I. McLoughlin, J.
    II. O'Boyle, P.J.
    [DNLM: 1. Urogenital
    System—surgery—handbooks.
    2. Surgery, Operative—methods—
    handbooks.
    WJ 39 T673   1995
    RD571. T66—1995
    617.4'6—dc20
    DNLM/DLC
    for Library of Congress

Contents

ENDOSCOPIC UROLOGY

Renal

Ureter

Bladder

Prostate

Urethra

Laparoscopy

Endoscopic equipment tips

OPEN UROLOGY

General points

Renal

Ureter

Bladder

Penis and scrotum

List of Contributors

P.D. Abel *Senior Lecturer and Honorary Consultant Urologist, Royal Postgraduate Medical School, Hammersmith Hospital, Du Cane Road, London W12 0NN*

D.G. Arkell *Consultant Urologist, Dudley Road Hospital, Dudley Road, Birmingham B18 7QH*

M.H. Ashken *Consultant Urologist, Norfolk and Norwich Hospital, Brunswick Road, Norwich NR1 3SR*

A.R.E. Blacklock *Consultant Urologist, Walsgrave Hospital, Clifford Bridge Road, Coventry CV2 2DX*

P.J.R. Boyd *Consultant Urologist, St Helier Hospital, Wrythe Lane, Carshalton, Surrey SM5 1AA*

K.N. Bullock *Consultant Urologist, Addenbrooke's Hospital, Hill's Road, Cambridge CB2 2QQ*

C.A.C. Charlton *Consultant Urologist, Royal United Hospital, Coombe Park, Bath BA2 7BR*

M.J. Coptcoat *Consultant Urologist, King's College Hospital, Denmark Hill, London SE5 9RS*

J. Cumming *Consultant Urologist, Southampton General Hospital, Tremona Road, Southampton SO9 4XY*

A.R. de Bolla *Consultant Urologist, Wrexham Maelor Hospital, Croesnewydd Road, Wrexham, Clwyd LL13 7TD*

I.K. Dickinson *Consultant Urologist, Joyce Green Hospital, Joyce Green Lane, Green Lane, Dartford, Kent DA1 5PL*

L.A. Emtage *Senior Registrar in Urology, Dudley Road Hospital, Birmingham B9 9JL*

R.C.L. Feneley *Consultant Urologist, Southmead Hospital, Westbury-on-Trym, Bristol BS10 5NB*

C.G. Fowler *Consultant Urologist, The Royal London Hospital, Whitechapel, London E1 1BB*

M. Fox *Consultant Urologist, Claremont Hospital, Sandygate Road, Sheffield, S10 5UB*

K.A. German *Senior Registrar in Urology, Edith Cavell Hospital, Bretton Gate, Peterborough PE3 9GZ*

N.O.K. Gibbon *Formerly Head of Urology Unit, Royal Liverpool Hospital, Prescott Street, Liverpool L7 8XP and Director of Urological Studies, Liverpool University*

H.W. Gilbert *Senior Registrar in Urology, Bristol Royal Infirmary, Marlborough Street, Bristol BS2 8HW*

J.C. Gingell *Consultant Urologist, Southmead Hospital, Westbury-on-Trym, Bristol BS10 5NB*

M.G.S. Golby *Consultant Urologist, Royal Devon and Exeter Hospital, Barrack Road, Exeter EX2 5DW*

W.F. Hendry *Consultant Urologist, St Bartholomew's Hospital, West Smithfield, London EC1A 7BE*

J.R. Hindmarsh *Consultant Urologist, South Cleveland Hospital, Marton Road, Middlesborough, Cleveland TS4 3BW*

J.H. Johnston *Formerly Consultant Urologist, Alderhay Children's Hospital, Eaton Road, West Derby L12 AP2 and Lecturer in Paediatric Urology, Liverpool University*

D.J. Jones *Consultant Urologist, Gloucestershire Royal Infirmary, Great Western Road, Gloucester GL1 3NN*

M.A. Jones *Consultant Urologist, Sandwell District Hospital, Lyndon, West Bromwich B71 4HJ*

J. Lawson *Consultant Surgeon, 149 Harley Street, London W1N 1HG*

R.J. Lemberger *Consultant Urologist, Nottingham City Hospital, Hucknall Road, Nottingham NG5 1PB*

R.J. Luck *Consultant Urologist, Wexham Park Hospital, Slough SL2 4H*

R.P. MacDonagh *Consultant Urologist, Musgrove Park Hospital, Taunton TA1 5DA*

J. McLoughlin *Consultant Urologist, West Suffolk Hospital, Hardwick Lane, Bury-St-Edmunds IP33 2QZ*

P.N. Matthews *Consultant Urologist, University Hospital of Wales, Heath Park, Cardiff CF4 4XW*

J.P. Mitchell *Honorary Professor of Surgery (Urology), Bristol University and Emeritus Consultant Urologist, United Bristol Hospitals and Southmead General Hospital, Bristol*

D.W.W. Newling *Professor of Urology, Academisch Ziekenhuis der Vrije Universiteit (AZUV), Postbus 7057, Amsterdam 1007 MB, The Netherlands*

R.G. Notley *Consultant Urologist, Royal Surrey County Hospital, Egerton Road, Guildford GU2 5XX*

F. Nuwayhid *Registrar in Urology, University Hospital of Wales, Heath Park, Cardiff CF4 4XW*

D.J. Oakland Formerly Consultant Urologist, Hereford County Hospital, Union Walk, Hereford HR1 2ER

P.J. O'Boyle Consultant Urologist, Musgrove Park Hospital, Taunton TA1 5DA

R.W.M. Rees Consultant Urologist, University Hospital of Wales, Heath Park, Cardiff CF4 4XW

A.B. Richards Consultant Urologist, The North Hampshire Hospital, Basingstoke RG24 9NA

A.N.S. Ritchie Consultant Urologist, Gloucestershire Royal Infirmary, Great Western Road, Gloucester GL1 3NN

J.C. Smith Consultant Urologist, Churchill Hospital, Old Road, Oxford OX3 7LJ

P.H. Smith Consultant Urologist, St James University Hospital, Great George Street, Leeds LS1 3EX

J.F. Somerville Consultant Urologist, Halifax General Hospital, Salterhebble, Halifax HX3 0PW

R.D.C. Southcott Consultant Urologist, Mayday Hospital, Thornton Health, Croydon CR7 7YE

M.J. Speakman Consultant Urologist, Musgrove Park Hospital, Taunton TA1 5DA

M.J. Stower Consultant Urologist, York District Hospital, Wiggington Road, York Y03 7HE

D.E. Sturdy Formerly Consultant General Surgeon and Urologist, Royal Gwent Hospital, Cardiff Road, Newport, Gwent NP9 2UB

G.C. Tresidder *Formerly Consultant Urologist, The Royal London Hospital, Whitechapel, London E1 1BB*

S.B.G. Vesey *Consultant Urologist, Southport and Formby District General Hospital, Town Lane, Kew, Southport PR8 6PH*

J. Vinnicombe *Consultant Urologist, St Mary's Hospital, Milton Road, Portsmouth PO6 3AD*

E.M. Walker *Consultant Urologist, Milton Keynes General Hospital, Standing Way, Eaglestone, Milton Keynes MK6 5LD*

A. Walsh *Consultant Urologist, 4 Donnybrook Close, Dublin 4, Ireland*

G.M. Watson *Consultant Urologist, Eastbourne District General Hospital, Kings Drive, Eastbourne BN21 2UD*

P.M.T. Weston *Consultant Urologist, Clayton Hospital, Northgate, Wakefield WF1 3JS*

R.H. Whitaker *Consultant Urologist, Addenbrooke's Hospital, Hill's Road, Cambridge CB2 2QQ*

J.A.K. Wightman *Formerly Consultant Urologist, The Royal Hospital, Chesterfield S44 5BL*

G. Williams *Consultant Urologist and Honorary Senior Lecturer, Royal Postgraduate Medical School, Hammersmith Hospital, Du Cane Road, London W12 0NN*

G.B. Williams *Consultant Urologist, Flat 3, 43 Wimpole Street, London W1M 7AB*

J.P. Williams *Formerly Consultant Urologist, St Peter's Hospital, Shaftesbury Avenue, London*

R.G. Willis *Consultant Urologist, Carlisle Hospitals NHS Trust, The Cumberland Infirmary, Newtown Road, Carlisle CA2 7HY*

R.O'N. Witherow *Consultant Urologist, St Mary's Hospital, Praed Street, London W2 1NY*

Foreword

All urologists have their favourite dodges and tricks to get around some of the technical problems and difficulties that might arise during operations and these can only be developed with experience, careful thought and sometimes courage to try out an idea that may have been born while in the bathtub. The weightier textbooks of urological surgery rarely can afford the space to tell you how to keep out of trouble during say, a radical prostatectomy, but it is precisely the desire to minimize unnecessary tachycardia and mopping of the brow that leads urologists to look for little ways to make the job easier for them and safer for the patient. Our surgical training is still based on apprenticeship and we learn new ways of operating from our teachers when we are registrars and from our colleagues when we take on consultant responsibility. However, there can be only a limited amount of exposure to this process, especially when a consultant. It is therefore, in my view, a brilliant concept to widen the field by gathering together in this little book ideas and experiences from so many urologists about their ways of dealing with various practical problems. While these may not be worthy of major articles in the journals, they can be like nuggets of gold to practising surgeons, especially those in training, and to young consultants.

W.B. Peeling
Royal Gwent Hospital
Newport, Gwent

Preface

At the heart of this book lie the little tricks and dodges which individual urologists use to either bail out from trouble, or to make a particular operation that little bit easier. Some you will have seen before and others will be new.

The book is based upon an imaginary situation where you have asked a senior colleague the question 'What do you do when?' or 'What if . . . happened?' The replies are by their very nature dogmatic and may not exactly conform to your own personal view. They have been kept as near to the original answers as possible in order to keep their flavour. The illustrations are based on simple line diagrams similar to those you would make on an operation record.

We hope that you will test the efficacy of these tips. No doubt you will let us know of any shortcomings and improvements which we can pass on to the authors who have entered into the spirit of this publication. We thank them all for their enthusiasm. On those rare occasions where two authors have offered tips of a similar nature both versions have been included in the text, albeit in an abbreviated form.

We hope you find it useful.

J. McLoughlin
P.J. O'Boyle

Acknowledgements

The authors are grateful for permission to reproduce the following illustrations:

Figure 11 from McLoughlin, J. (1994) *British Journal of Urology* **74**, 118.

Figure 31 from Gepi-Attee, S., Ganabathi, K. and Gingell, J.C. (1990) *British Journal of Urology* **66**, 439–440.

Figure 33 from Frank, J.D. and Johnston, J.H. (eds) (1990) *Operative Paediatric Urology*. Churchill Livingstone, Edinburgh.

Figure 36 from Notley, R.G. and Thomson, A.A.G. (1978) *Journal of Urology* **120**, 159–161.

Figure 39 from Hendry, W.F., Christmas, T.J. and Shepherd, J.H. (1991) *Journal of the Royal Society of Medicine* **84**, 709–712.

Figure 49 from Gilroy-Bevan, P. (ed.) (1982) *Reconstructive Procedures in Surgery*. Blackwell Scientific Publications, Oxford.

Figure 50 from Fox, M. (1994) *British Journal of Urology* **73**, 449–453.

Figure 51 from Joseph, M.J. and O'Boyle, P.J. (1989) *Journal of the Royal College of Surgeons of Edinburgh* **34**, 104–105.

Figure 52 from McLoughlin, J. and O'Boyle, P.J. (1994) *British Journal of Urology* **74**, 515.

Endoscopic Urology

Renal

Access for percutaneous renal procedures
J. Cumming

For those of us who provide their own access to the renal collecting system, I have found this tip reduces the failure rate of access. At the stage where the patient is semi-prone with a ureteric catheter inserted retrogradely, radiographic contrast is usually employed to identify the collecting system. If multiple punctures are made in order to find the optimal point of entry, the contrast may start to leak out and fog the picture of the image intensifier.

My tip is to use air which gives a good outline of the collecting system. Pump a little diluted methylene blue dye (only) up the retrograde catheter and blue-tinged bubbles may be seen when the trochar is withdrawn from the needle. I rarely use liquid contrast which has the added advantage of avoiding rare allergic reactions (1 : 30 000) and cost.

Percutaneous nephrolithotomy
A.N.S. Ritchie and H.W. Gilbert

When the renal cortex is thickened or the kidney is mobile, the progressive dilatation of a percutaneous nephrolithotomy track with telescopic bougies can become arrested when a bougie fails to penetrate the renal cortex. This impass is easily overcome by the passage of an optical urethrotome blade over the number 2 bougie. The blade is guided down to the renal cortex where a small incision can be made, if necessary, under X-ray screening (Fig. 1). The remaining bougies will then pass with ease.

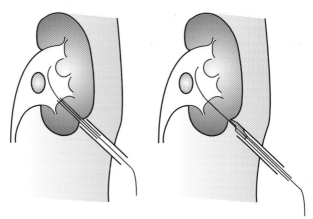

Figure 1

Percutaneous nephrolithotomy
R.G. Willis

We carry this out in one stage in theatre and pass a (balloon) ureteric catheter first in order to fill the collecting system with contrast mixed with methylene blue. Sometimes, despite what looks like a promising track dilatation, when you introduce the nephroscope you find you are either not quite in the collecting system or are through the other side! Sometimes, the guide wire is not quite where it ought to be and also leads you astray—*merde*!

My tip is that if you are just a little lost like this, ask an assistant to inject methylene blue again via the ureteric catheter and look for a jet of blue dye emerging from the parenchyma. Once seen, follow the blue jet with your nephroscope and you can often re-enter the collecting system and retrieve the situation.

Flexible ureterorenoscopy
M.J. Coptcoat

The indications for retrograde flexible ureterorenoscopy are limited to the diagnosis of small filling defects, coupled with the sight of haematuria, when more usual forms of imaging have been inconclusive, or the endoscopic fragmentation of a small renal stone that has proved to be recalcitrant to extracorporeal shockwave lithotripsy, and is not suitable for percutanous nephrolithotomy. One cannot underestimate the difficulty of passing even the smallest calibre instruments all the way up to the kidney unless the preliminary procedures are followed.

I find it almost mandatory to insert a double J stent for 48 h. This produces a mild dilatation effect but more importantly increases the compliance of the ureter. The double J stent is removed at 48 h and under a general anaesthetic a

6 F catheter with side holes is passed up to the kidney. This catheter allows a continuous flow of irrigation during passage of the flexible endoscope that would otherwise cause a local high pressure situation and immediate retrograde absorption of fluid, with a possible danger of septicaemia. A peel-away sheath is then placed into the ureteric orifice leaving the ureteric catheter on the outside. The flexible ureterorenoscope can then be passed over a 0.025 inch guide wire up to the kidney. High pressure irrigation is useful during its retrograde passage, but once the kidney is reached, the guide wire can be removed and irrigation can be continued at low pressure. All subsequent manoeuvres within the kidney should be monitored on an image intensifier to maintain the correct orientation.

These steps are not always needed and there is the occasional patient, in particular a multiparous female, where the flexible ureterorenoscope can be passed at the first attempt with no preliminary dilatation and without any sheath. However, if the above steps are followed, retrograde flexible ureteroscopy can be a safe and successful procedure every time.

Ureter

Easy introduction of the rigid ureteroscope
K.N. Bullock

Many methods of dilating the ureteric orifice to allow the introduction of a rigid ureteroscope have been described. The most common cause of failure is inability to introduce the instrument into the ureteric orifice.

One irrigation channel of the ureteroscope should be connected to a standard irrigation bag of saline as normal. The second port is connected to a 1 litre bag of saline, pressurized to maximum pressure with a Fenwell bag. Once the ureteroscope has been inserted into the bladder a Pfister–Schwarz or Segura basket is passed along the instrument channel into the ureteric orifice before the instrument is introduced (Fig. 2).

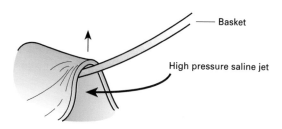

Figure 2

The high pressure irrigation is switched on and the normal irrigation off. The ureteroscope is then inverted before insertion into the ureteric orifice. Inversion allows the basket to tent the roof of the ureteric orifice upwards and the high pressure splays open the orifice, allowing easy introduction of the ureteroscope. Using this technique, an 11 F ureteroscope can be readily introduced into the orifice without significant trauma under direct vision.

Once the intramural ureter has been traversed, the high pressure irrigation is closed and normal irrigation restarted to prevent blowing stones back into the kidney. The stone basket is then already in position as a guide to further insertion of the instrument and can be opened immediately to snare any stone visualized.

Pressure over the abdominal wall helps pass a ureteroscope
G.M. Watson

The ureter is attached to the posterior peritoneum, and it passes over muscles and vessels in the retroperitoneum. It is surprising, therefore, that pressure over the abdominal wall at a level approximating to the tip of the ureteroscope can influence the position of the ureter immediately above the ureteroscope (Fig. 3). If faced with a tortuous ureter, use a video camera if possible. Request that the patient has an anaesthetic with full muscle relaxation. Have the height of the table at waist level. Place a hand over the abdomen level with the tip of the ureteroscope, then search for the position over which abdominal pressure brings the ureter ahead into alignment. This is most helpful when attempting to negotiate the iliac vessels at the pelvic brim. If trying to get into the upper third then pressure by an assistant under the loin can again straighten the ureter.

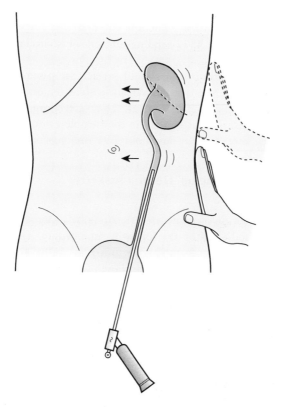

Figure 3

Ureteroscopy for stones
R.G. Willis

Do not waste time trying to extract ureteric stones intact. Use an electrohydraulic lithotriptor (carefully) to break the stone into many pieces and, via the ureteroscope, pass a ureteric catheter up to the kidney. Secure the ureteric catheter so that it drains *into* a latex Foley catheter using the Raper method*. Get on with the next case on your list and remove both the Foley and the ureteric catheter from the patient after 48 h, sending him or her home later that day.

If you feel you can or should extract the stone, I sometimes use the Microvasive Macaluso stent-removing three-pronged 4.5 F grasping forceps. They are cheap, are very good for fishing out stents via the flexible cystoscope and are also very effective down our 9.5 F ureteroscope.

'Two down–one up' Dormia basketry
J. McLoughlin

The extraction of a low ureteric stone by a Dormia basket can be facilitated by the following manoeuvre. This technique was shown to me by Mr Smith at the Bristol Royal Infirmary, but owes its origin to the original description by Dormia. Pass the fully collapsed basket up the ureter for 2–3 cm beyond the stone. The basket is then opened fully and gently retrieved and re-inserted alternately — two gradations out followed by one gradation back in. No attempt should be made to close the basket. Instead, the two down–one up movement allows the stone to 'roll along' in front of the basket. Once the stone has been pulled half out of the ureteric orifice the basket can be closed to allow the stone to be secured before it falls into the bladder.

---

* The method of securing a ureteric catheter described by F. Raper (formerly of Leeds) is simply to use a number 11 scalpel blade to pierce the connecting funnel of a latex Foley catheter and push the ureteric catheter's end through into the lumen of the Foley.

The Sachse urethrotome
E.M. Walker

The Sachse urethrotome is an excellent instrument for extraction of ureteric calculi. Its square cut end makes the passage of the basket via its instrument channel into the ureteric orifice easy. It comes into its element when a stone is stuck in the basket in the intra-mural ureter and will not budge. The knife blade can be passed alongside the stone under direct vision and either used to spade the stone sideways or, if this is unsuccessful, it can be used to make a small controlled cut in the ureteric orifice and so ease the passage of the stone into the bladder.

Using the pusher first technique to facilitate the insertion of a double J stent
P.J. O'Boyle

Open-ended double J stents require the initial passage of a flexible tipped guide wire, along which the stent is then rail-roaded. It can prove very difficult to direct the guide wire into the ureteric orifice — the end of the wire can fall off the deflecting mechanism.

By inserting the pusher *first* this effectively produces a tunnel guide which can be positioned either immediately adjacent to the ureteric orifice, or at any desired position in relation to it. The guide wire is then inserted through the inner lumen of the pusher and up to the ureteric orifice (Fig. 4, p. 12). Following wire placement, the pusher can be withdrawn and used in the usual manner to push home the double J stent.

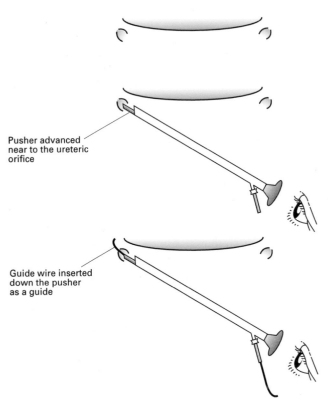

Figure 4

Double J stenting

G.B. Williams

When placing double J stents, the 'pusher' sometimes fails to disengage from the stent when you take out the guide wire. Advance the pusher as you withdraw the cystoscope: 2 cm in on the pusher and 2 cm out with the cystoscope. As the cystoscope beak emerges from the external urethral meatus, grasp the pusher and deliver it from the cystoscope.

Now, with the cystoscope alongside the 'pusher', change the 30° telescope for the 'cup' biopsy forceps with a 30° or 0° telescope and grasp the lower end of the stent. Do not grasp too hard or you will transect it. When you have a firm grip on the stent with the biopsy forceps, just pull out the 'pusher'.

Securing ureteric catheters
S.B.G. Vesey

Ureteric catheters inserted in the operating theatre frequently become dislodged while patients are transported to the X-ray department for retrograde pyelography. This simple technique, learned at Musgrove Park Hospital, Taunton, has been found to be very satisfactory for safely securing ureteric catheters during transportation.

Following insertion of the ureteric catheter, a latex Foley balloon catheter is inserted per urethram. The inflated balloon is drawn down onto the bladder neck. A ureteric catheter is piggy-backed into the connecting end of the Foley catheter by threading it over an 18 G needle passed outwards from within the lumen of the catheter (Fig. 5a, p. 14). This not only secures the ureteric catheter but it also allows its free drainage when a urinary drainage bag is attached to the Foley catheter.

A tidy method for ureteric catheters
L.A. Emtage

Sending patients from the operating threatre to the X-ray department with a ureteric catheter is made easy and neat by nicking the urethral catheter with a scalpel blade just enough to allow the entry of the ureteric catheter into the widened connecting lumen of the catheter (Fig. 5b, p. 14). The small catheter can be further splinted using tape to

(a)

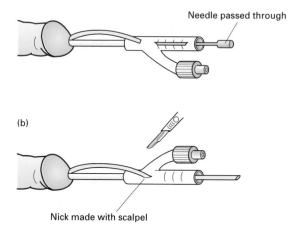

Needle passed through

(b)

Nick made with scalpel

Figure 5

attach it to the urethral catheter. This avoids separate containers which often become disconnected when the patient is moved. Manipulation of the tip of the ureteric catheter is easy as it can be flipped out to be connected to a syringe for the retrograde study.

Ureteric catheters

R.O'N. Witherow

This simple method allows a retrograde catheter to be kept sterile. An urethral catheter is placed and the retrograde is taped to it to prevent it being dislodged. A number 11 blade is passed from inside the drainage channel of the urethral catheter, approximately 1 cm from the end. When the tip protrudes through the wall, the end of the retrograde catheter is pushed over this and penetrates inside the drainage channel of the urethral catheter (Fig. 5b). The retrograde catheter is then fed inside the channel of the drainage bag where it can drain freely, and remains sterile until any further procedure is carried out.

How to prevent guide wires, Dormia baskets and ureteric extras from leaping off the trolley onto the floor
P.J. O'Boyle

Quite often ureteroscopic accessories are difficult to control when lying on a theatre trolley. They can be kept firmly in place by fixing two towel clips about 0.5 m apart and using the loops created by the jaws of the forceps as grips. Flexible guide wires can also be subdued in the same way by making a loop of the guide wire and returning it back through the handle of one of the forceps (Fig. 6).

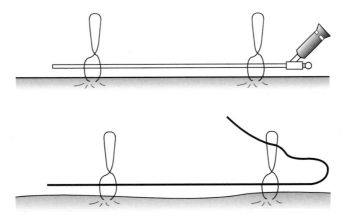

Figure 6

Use of the ureteric catheter sheath to prevent contamination of the ureteric catheter

P.J. O'Boyle

Ureteric catheters come conveniently packed in tubular sheaths. Usually, these are discarded when the catheter is loaded on the trolley . . . what folly! The tube container is ideal to prevent contamination of the catheter during early manipulation when the catheter is prone to flail about. For those unfortunates who do not have a microvideo operating system this usually results in the catheter brushing against one's face.

Leave the catheter in its rigid container, permitting only 2.5 cm to protrude before introducing it into the deflecting mechanism. The ureteric catheter can then be introduced still sterile, having been protected by the external sleeve. Moreover, if the initial manoeuvre is unsuccessful the catheter can be withdrawn back into the rigid sheath which is much less vulnerable to displacement on the frequently cluttered operating trolley.

Bladder

Risks in the use of spinal anaesthesia for the resection of bladder tumours
D.W.W. Newling

The resection of tumours on the anterior wall and vault of the bladder is made very much easier if the patient can be placed in an exaggerated Trendelenburg position. With the increasing use of spinal anaesthesia this is frequently not possible, making the resection both more difficult and probably incomplete if the tumour is of considerable size. I found it extremely useful to acquaint the anaesthetist with the position of the tumour in this respect, prior to his or her decision on the type of anaesthesia that will be used.

Bladder diverticulas
G.B. Williams

Operating on a bladder diverticulum as an open procedure must be close to black magic — you cannot prove anything! However, when the bladder diverticulum is present when *resecting* superficial bladder tumours how do you know 'they' are not in the diverticulum now, or in the future?

Transurethral quadrantic incision of the neck of the diverticulum with a Colling's knife electrode down to the perivesical fat dramatically opens up the diverticulum (Fig. 7, p. 18). Change the Colling's electrode for a ball electrode and destroy the urothelium of the diverticulum with it. Leave a catheter in for 3 days. A check cystoscopy 3 months later shows the diverticulum has gone. If you are worried about the ureter adjacent put a ureteric catheter up the ureter first.

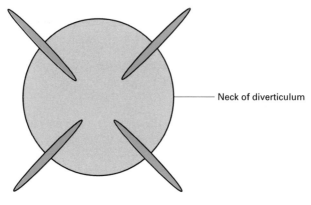

Neck of diverticulum

Figure 7

Resection of vault and posterior wall bladder tumours
K.A. German

The resection of tumours situated on the posterior wall and vault of the bladder can be awkward. I was given this tip by Reg Hall who advised leaving the loop extended and swinging the whole resectoscope in an arc rather than drawing in the loop in the conventional manner.

Using a balanced irrigation system, the cutting diathermy is started *before* contact is made with the bladder mucosa. In a slow and deliberate manner the resectoscope is swung in one direction in a side-to-side arc resecting the tumour with cutting diathermy active the whole time (Fig. 8). This manoeuvre reduces the potential for bladder perforation because, as the direction of resection is maintained parallel with the contour of the bladder wall, the operator can proceed with a much better control of the depth of resection.

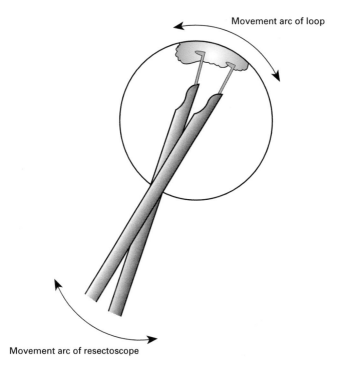

Movement arc of loop

Movement arc of resectoscope

Figure 8

That elusive stone or chip
D.G. Arkell

A most useful and speedy way to remove that elusive small stone, prostate chip or blood clot from the bladder which has defied even the Ellick's evacuator is to employ the 'suction effect' of a cystoscope or resectoscope. Position the end of the sheath's beak directly on to the fragment, stop the flow of irrigant and then quickly remove the telescope from it sheath. Angle the sheath downwards and the fragment is usually retrieved when the residual fluid in the bladder is emptied.

Removing stone fragments using the stone punch
J. McLoughlin

Using the Storz stone punch to break up bladder calculi can be tedious and frustrating if either the bladder capacity is reduced, or even a minor amount of bleeding is encountered as this tends to obscure the view.

My tip is to forget trying to use the outflow channel of the stone punch at all. Instead, simply turn on, and leave on, the inflow channel. As soon as you have a stone (or fragment) in the jaws of the punch, close the jaws and extract the inner element with the stone trapped inside, keeping the sheath still in relation to the urethra. The bladder will then partially empty in the few seconds it takes to remove the fragment from the jaws. It is important to retrieve the fragments through the sheath. (The practice of jamming the larger fragments against the end of the sheath and removing the whole ensemble with the stone snatched onto the end is dangerous and can result in urethral tears. It is better to spend a little time reducing the stone fragment size.) Repeat the process. You will need a scrub nurse with a kidney dish nearby to avoid getting soaked.

While it may sound slow it is actually surprisingly fast as you always have irrigant clearing your view in much the same way that you would with a continuous flow resectoscope, and pretty soon you are left with a few small fragments which can be evacuated with the Ellick's.

This same technique can be used for finishing off the fragments that remain, having broken up larger stones with the lithoclast/electrohydraulic probe.

Avoiding disaster with the lithotrite

R.C.L. Feneley and R.P. MacDonagh

The Storz optical lithotrite (2707A) is invaluable for crush-ing bladder stones, but it can present the surgeon with a horrific problem if the jaws become dislocated within the bladder during use. Legendary tales exist of surgeons who have opened the bladder to release the blades of the lithotrite or who have ordered a hacksaw to divide the instrument into two halves.

The jaws of the lithotrite can dislocate if it is incorrectly assembled. There are two screws (Fig. 9, points 1 and 2) on the upper border of the instrument which must be tight-ened to ensure that the inner and outer jaws are correctly retained and aligned. Failure to check these screws before introducing the instrument can lead to dislocation of the jaws and an alarming experience for the surgeon if unpre-pared for such an eventuality. Under such circumstances, no attempt should be made to remove the instrument tran-surethrally. The following procedure should be observed to dismantle and remove the instrument.

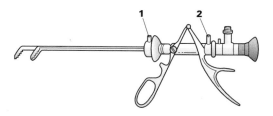

Figure 9

Firstly, remove the telescope, turn off the taps and dis-connect the irrigation set but leave the bladder full. Unscrew the two screws on the upper border of the shaft and then remove the handle of the instrument, by holding the shaft of the jaws and pulling the handle straight back.

The two holes on the shaft of the jaws, which hold the tips of the screws when the lithotrite is fully assembled, should then be carefully aligned. The inner shaft should be gently pulled back, clicking in position if the alignment of the holes has been maintained, exposing an engraved rail. This will confirm that the jaws are properly closed. Ensure that the jaws are retained in the closed position, rotate the shaft until the holes point posteriorly in relation to the patient and remove the shaft in the usual manner for a beaked instrument.

Although the lithoclast and the Storz Mauermayer stone punch (27077A/B) may be preferred instruments for stone destruction, there is still a place for the optical lithotrite. Any surgeon would be well advised to learn how to reassemble the lithotrite before using the instrument.

Day case cystoscopy
R.C.L. Feneley

When undertaking day case cystoscopy under general anaesthesia, I always ask the anaesthetist to give 20 mg frusemide intravenously at the end of the procedure. This results in the patient voiding good volumes soon after the examination and ensures that when you see your patients after the list you can be sure they have passed urine.

Bladder biopsies
J.P. Williams

In cases of interstitial cystitis plus a thin-walled bladder, if you propose doing a biopsy in conjunction with a hydrostatic dilatation, remember to perform the biopsy after, not before, the dilatation, lest a dark cavern be seen and it will not be a day case . . . (I need hardly say, need I, that this happened to somebody else).

Flexible cystoscopy
M.J. Stower

With the rapid turnover of a flexible cystoscope list it is often difficult to get urine cytology when perhaps one should. Nurses often forget to collect it when the patient voids before the cystoscopy. I have found that if you take the tap off the flexible cystoscope and attach a 10 ml syringe when there is some irrigant in the bladder one can obtain a perfectly adequate sample for cytology.

Flexible cystoscopy
M.J. Stower

In men, I have found that if you get someone to squeeze the irrigation bag while you are passing a flexible cystoscope the patient experiences much less discomfort, in particular when you are easing through the sphincters.

Placement of the difficult suprapubic catheter
D.J. Jones

This technique was taught by Richard Turner-Warwick at the Institute of Urology and is useful for inserting a suprapubic catheter into a small contracted bladder which will not dilate sufficiently with fluid to allow accurate localization, or in an obese patient when the bladder cannot be easily palpated or percussed.

Under general anaesthetic or regional anaesthetic, a preliminary cystoscopy is first performed. A 14 Ch Hay–Groves dilator, which has been customized by drilling a hole 0.5 cm from the tip, is passed into the bladder and the anterior wall tented up suprapubically (Fig. 10). An incision is made onto the tip of the dilator which is then advanced through the abdominal wall. A Foley catheter of the desired size is tied to the dilator using the catheter eye and drill hole. The dilator and catheter are then withdrawn from the bladder and out of the urethra. The tie is divided and the catheter carefully withdrawn back into the bladder, inflating the balloon gently as it passes through the urethra. Although Bonano suprapubic catheters and Nottingham

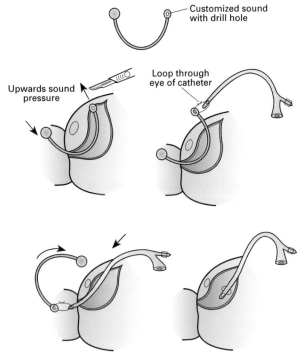

Customized sound with drill hole

Upwards sound pressure

Loop through eye of catheter

Figure 10

introducers will be appropriate for most placements, this technique is invaluable in 'awkward' bladders.

Siting of the suprapubic catheter
A.R.E. Blacklock

In females, pass a closed cholecystectomy or similar forceps up the urethra. Angle the forceps so that the closed points are palpable as the anterior bladder wall is tented up underneath the anterior abdominal wall in the suprapubic region. Cut down onto the point of the forceps with a small scalpel, incising until the point of the forceps can be pushed through the skin incision. Next, open the forceps and grasp a suitably sized Foley catheter by its tip and pull into the bladder and out along the urethra. The balloon of the catheter can be slowly inflated as the catheter is drawn back into the bladder so that the inflated balloon lies in the bladder. The final position can be checked with a cystoscope.

In males, pass urethrally a curved metal bougie, such as a Lister's, of equal size or one size larger than the catheter to be inserted. Tent up the anterior bladder wall as previously described and cut down on the bougie so that the bougie can be pushed out through the suprapubic skin incision. Tie the tip of the catheter to the tip of the bougie with any suitable ligature material, aligning the tip of the catheter adjacent to the tip of the bougie. Pull the catheter into the bladder and along the urethra as before. Cut the tie and pull the catheter back into the bladder, gently inflating the balloon so that the fully inflated balloon lies in the bladder. Finally, check its position with a cystoscope.

Tying the knot during a Stamey colposuspension
J. McLoughlin

If plastic tubing is used as a buttress for the rectus sheath component of the Stamey colposuspension the knot tends to slip, so that optimal tension is not maintained. Also, the knot displaces the tubing downwards so that it lies awkwardly against the sheath. The technique is a simple means of ensuring that not only does the buttress remain aligned, but also that it imparts a degree of resistance in the knot, permitting the surgeon to maintain optimal tension while completing the knot.

The buttress (size 8 F infant feeding tube) is threaded over one end of the suture and two throws are gently made (Fig. 11). The suture end adjacent to the buttress is then also passed through, after which the remaining throws are made to complete the knot.

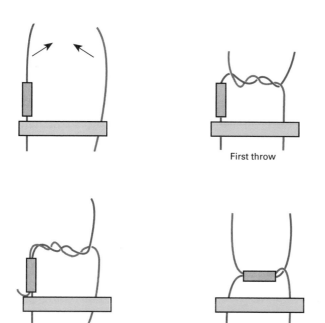

First throw

Thread the end
through the buttress

Push down on the buttress
with the index finger whilst
pulling on either end

Throw a second time
and secure the knot

Figure 11

Prostate

Golby's gallows
M.G.S. Golby

The illustration (Fig. 12) shows a simple aid to suspend the fibre-optic light cable and fluid tubing from above the patient on the operating table while performing a transurethral resection of the prostate. It stops getting everything in a knot and the equipment is easy to obtain.

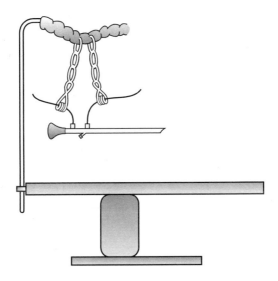

Figure 12

A 1.25 cm chromium-plated rod 2 m long is bent to a right angle 0.5 m from its top with a small concave dip 15 cm from the top end. This can be fixed to the side of the operating table by a standard bracket, the top end being covered by a

0.5 m length of anaesthetic tubing stapled closed at one end. Six thick elastic bands linked together have a chromium-plated spiral loop attached to either end and hang over the support at the point where the anaesthetic tubing-covered rod assumes a concave dip.

The anaesthetic tubing, elastic bands and loop are sterilized before use. The sterile light cable and fluid tubing are threaded through the loops and hand down on springs.

Gibbon's hook
P.J. O'Boyle

The famous golfing urologist N.O.K. Gibbon is remembered not only for his exaggerated fading of the golf ball but also for a very simple and inexpensive device which has saved many a telescope from plunging to an untimely fate.

A simple steel malleable tube is covered with antistatic rubber and bent at each end into a hook. It can then be conveniently suspended from the theatre light and positioned immediately above the patient. The light lead, irrigation tubing, diathermy lead and camera lead are gathered together by two interlocking stout elastic bands and suspended from the lower hook. The theatre light can be adjusted to take the weight of the resectoscope and attachments. This also keeps the leads tidy and, particularly in the female, should the resectoscope slide out of the urethra while unattended it is left suspended above the patient rather than crashing into the effluent bin or worse.

Bilateral bladder neck incisions facilitate the resection of large median lobes
J. McLoughlin

This useful manoeuvre was shown to me by Paddy O'Boyle of Taunton. One of the problems with large median lobes is the tendency to undermine the bladder neck when resecting it. Bilateral incisions at 5 and 7 o'clock using the Colling's knife allow the median lobe to drop and also enables one to define the position of the bladder neck fibres on either side of the median lobe prior to resection.

The undercut
J.R. Hindmarsh

The sequence of resection during prostatectomy will vary from case to case, but each surgeon through time and habit will more or less acquire a set pattern of resection after his or her first thousand transurethral resections.

I always found bleeding from the bladder neck, prostatic base and alongside the veru troublesome until I realized that by resecting the bladder neck followed by taking three or four full-length chips (bladder neck to veru) from the lowest part of each lateral lobe resulted in a wide cavity. This allows the troublesome vessels from the bladder neck to the veru to be easily visible and quickly diathermized at that time (Fig. 13). In addition, the prostatic lateral lobes prolapse easily into the urethra leading to rapid resection. Once the prostatic urethra has been dealt with in this way, which takes 2–3 min, there is no need to return to it and the bleeding is secured. This operation is locally known as the 'kindest undercut of all'.

Transurethral resection of the prostate (TURP)
J.F. Somerville

At the end of a TURP, bring the resectoscope distal to the veru to inspect the resection at the apex of the prostate. It is surprising how often one finds quite large tags of prostatic tissue that have been left behind and need to be resected. Everyone may already be doing this! No one ever suggested it to me and I have only recently started doing it.

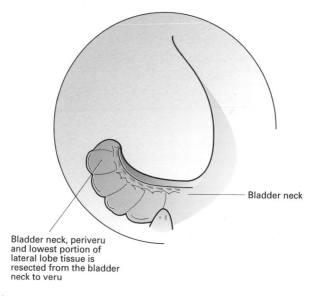

Bladder neck

Bladder neck, periveru
and lowest portion of
lateral lobe tissue is
resected from the bladder
neck to veru

Figure 13

Haemostasis after transurethral resection of the prostate
R.J. Lemberger

If the glycine infusion rate is slowed right down this makes all bleeders much more obvious, presumably because the high flow rate washes the blood so quickly into the bladder that some vessels are not visible. The flow rate can be turned down while looking and it is obvious when to stop reducing it further. This certainly enhances haemostasis.

Transurethral resection of the prostate (TURP)
P.D. Abel

I like to fill the bladder after a TURP, before removing the resectoscope and after having washed out. If there is any difficulty then in getting the bladder catheterized, you have a little time to either sort it out or replace the resectoscope and see what the problem is without there being too much clotting off.

Dealing with torrential bleeding from the prostate
G.M. Watson

Richard Turner-Warwick told me this one for severe bleeding from the prostate or bladder that is not controlled by conventional techniques. Pass ureteric catheters up both ureters. Open the bladder in the coronal plane (as one would for a clam cystoplasty). Exchange single J catheters for the ureteric catheters and bring the single J catheters out through the anterior abdominal wall. Then, suture the anterior wall of the bladder to the posterior wall using 0 dexon or chromic catgut. The sutures start at the trigone and then come progressively to the vault. This tamponades the bladder. A bleeding prostate is also controlled. Six weeks later the J stents can be removed and the patient will have a near normal capacity because the sutures will have dissolved.

The management of clot retention
R.C.L. Feneley

The urgent management of the patient with clot retention of urine can be a daunting task for the inexperienced clinician. Evacuation of the clot is essential and adequate drainage of the bladder should then be established.

A Foley-type catheter with a self-retaining balloon does not have a sufficiently wide internal lumen to allow the clots to be readily aspirated with a bladder syringe. There is virtually always far more clot than anticipated and a wide-bore catheter is required. A 24 F or 26 F Harris catheter provides a reasonable internal lumen to aspirate clots from the bladder. Irrigation and aspiration with a 60 ml syringe of sterile water or saline solution should enable the operator to evacuate the bladder of clots. If the bleeding continues following the aspiration, it is prude to strap the catheter into the bladder rather than exchange it for a self-retaining balloon catheter (Fig. 14).

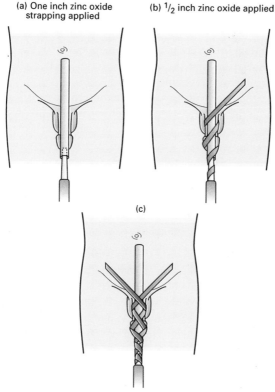

(a) One inch zinc oxide strapping applied

(b) ¹/₂ inch zinc oxide applied

(c)

Figure 14

1 Shave the lower abdomen and suprapubic region. I recommend using 1 inch and 0.5 inch zinc oxide tape to strap the catheter into the bladder. Adjust the catheter so that the tip is lying within the bladder and is draining freely.

2 Run a length of 1 inch zinc oxide strapping from just below the umbilicus in the midline down to and along the dorsum of the penis onto the catheter for about 3.5–5 cm and mould the strapping around the catheter (Fig. 14a).

3 Next, run a length of 0.5 inch zinc oxide strapping from the medial side of the anterior superior iliac spine obliquely down to the dorsum of the penis, then spiral it around the penis for two or three turns before passing it onto the catheter (Fig. 14b). Repeat the same manoeuvre for the opposite side starting from the medial aspect of the contralateral anterior superior iliac spine (Fig. 14c).

The catheter provides a satisfactory intermittent irrigation system. In the early days of transurethral surgery this system was used routinely for all prostate operations in Bristol in conjunction with the two-way irrigation system which incorporated a Higginson-type rubber syringe.

Control of venous bleeding following transurethral resection of the prostate
F. Nuwayhid and P.N. Matthews

On occasions, all urologists face the difficulty of controlling venous bleeding following a transurethral prostatectomy. Traction to tamponade bleeding can be achieved by applying continuous pressure from several strong elastic bands (Fig. 15). Sustained 'safe' traction can be applied for several hours if necessary but should be released for 10 min each hour. This type of traction is simple to perform, quick to apply and easy for the nurse to manage.

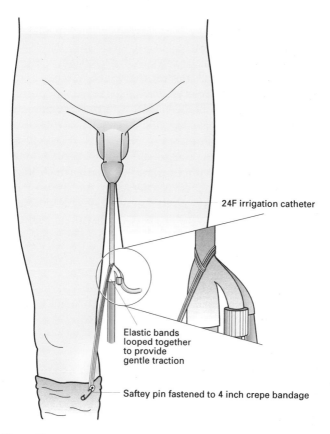

24F irrigation catheter

Elastic bands
looped together
to provide
gentle traction

Saftey pin fastened to 4 inch crepe bandage

Figure 15

Haemorrhage after retropubic prostatectomy
R.G. Willis

Avoid the temptation to re-open the wound. On return to theatre for bleeding follow these steps.

1 Insert your largest resectoscope.

2 Thoroughly wash out the bladder with an Ellick.

3 Use the resectoscope loop 'cold' to sweep forwards all the clots from the prostatic cavity.

4 Further wash out the bladder and prostatic cavity.

5 Use the roller ball to coagulate everything which might bleed, especially around the bladder neck.

In this way, you can probably secure excellent haemostasis without re-opening a very ill patient and without resort to the dreaded packing. It is better to strike early rather than wait until the eighth unit of blood!

Urethra

The fractured pelvis and the 'S' bend urethra
J.P. Mitchell

Every urologist at some time must have been faced with the problem of a patient with multiple injuries including a fractured pelvis, who must go to theatre without delay for some uncontrolled bleeding. The general surgeon wishes to know as soon as possible whether the patient also has a ruptured urethra. There is insufficient time to wait for the bladder to fill, and no urologist today would rely on the 'diagnostic' catheter.

Nothing is lost by a quick, but very gentle, urethroscopy performed by an experienced endoscopist as soon as the patient is anaesthetized. This will clearly reveal any damage to the urethral mucosa or urethral wall. Occasionally, bleeding is too heavy to obtain a good view, but surely then there can be no doubt about urethral trauma. Even mucosal damage without a complete rupture of the wall of the urethra will heal with less risk of stricture formation if a suprapubic urinary diversion is performed and left for 10–14 days.

The endoscopist must beware of the 'S' bend deformity in the posterior urethra (Fig. 16, p. 38) due to backward displacement of the proximal segment of the urethra by the fractured pelvis and by infrapubic haematoma. The 'S' bend can deceive the unwary, resulting in either iatrogenic trauma to the anterior wall of the urethra from the tip of the endoscope (Fig. 16a), or missing a small rupture in the posterior aspect of the urethral wall just beyond the 'S' bend, where the urethra may be obscured unless the instrument is tilted specifically to view this area (Fig. 16b).

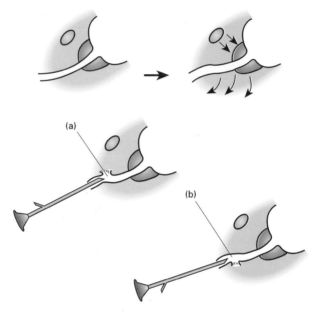

Figure 16

How to use an Otis urethrotome in an awkward urethra

G.M. Watson

Richard Turner-Warwick showed me this trick. The end of the Otis urethrotome is slightly bulbous. This can be detached by unscrewing to reveal an underlying screw thread. Pass a 6 F ureteric catheter through the stricture and then screw the ureteric catheter onto the screw thread at the end of the Otis. Follow the ureteric catheter with the Otis as one would with a filiform and follower. The urethrotome can then be passed into the bladder and one can dilate the urethra using the urethrotome blade.

Getting through an 'impassable' urethral stricture
C.G. Fowler

It is sometimes impossible to find a way through an urethral stricture using instruments passed retrogradely. In the past, it used to be necessary to perform a formal cystotomy and pass instruments from above to find the way. The modern way to do this is as follows.

Make sure the bladder is full. Make a stab suprapubic cystotomy using Will Lawrence's suprapubic catheter introducer (Femcare). This is just large enough to allow a standard Olympus CYF-2 flexible cystoscope to pass retrogradely into the bladder and thence into the urethra (Fig. 17, p. 40). It is sometimes possible to pass a guide wire through the stricture from above. If not, turn off the light to the optical urethrotome and cut towards the red glow from the 'headlights' of the flexible cystoscope.

The difficult urethral stricture
J.P. Mitchell

A patient with a difficult or apparently impassable urethral stricture presents a problem easily solved if he or she also has a suprapubic cystotomy, as may be present when a temporary urinary diversion has been performed for a fractured pelvis with urethral damage.

A flexible endoscope passed into the bladder down to the internal urethral meatus and then down the proximal urethra can provide a light source which will be visible via the endoscopic urethrotome passed from below towards the stricture face. The site to cut with the urethrotome knife will then clearly be obvious. If no transmitted light can be seen then either the proximal endoscope is not in the urethra or there has been gross disruption of the urethral alignment and not just a simple stricture.

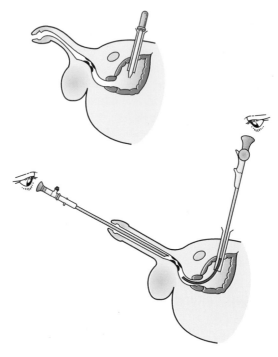

Figure 17

Catheter introducers

J.A.K. Wightman

Catheter introducers are frequently not of much help in passing urethral catheters since they are flexible, often deformed by previous use and sometimes difficult to extract from the interior of the catheter once it has been introduced into the bladder. In addition, the wide curve and flexible nature of the tip makes it difficult to judge the correct track into the bladder.

To overcome this problem a number 6/10 sound, introduced into the eye of a Foley catheter and then well lubricated, serves the purpose much better in that the introducing instrument is rigid, has a curve which one is used to using to negotiate the posterior urethra and the sound is easily extracted once the catheter balloon has been deflated (Fig. 18).

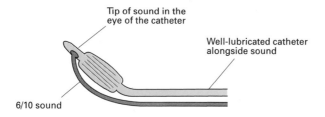

Tip of sound in the eye of the catheter

Well-lubricated catheter alongside sound

6/10 sound

Figure 18

The Maryfield introducer
R.D.C. Southcott

Use the Maryfield (exterior) catheter introducer, medium size, and throw away all those wire things! The channel between the catheter and introducer should be thoroughly lubricated. The catheter can be disengaged either by advancing it as the introducer is withdrawn or by gently inflating the balloon which forces the tip of the introducer out of the catheter eye.

Laparoscopy

Introduction of the first port for laparoscopy
M.J. Coptcoat

Hasson described a technique for the open introduction of the first port for laparoscopy*. This is a simple technique that requires an incision of only 2 cm, but carries with it a guarantee of safe insertion of the cannula every time into the peritoneal cavity. A Hasson blunt-tipped port is designed for use when adopting this approach. This is especially useful when a patient may have adhesions from previous surgery or when the laparoscopic surgeon has less experience.

*Editorial note: a small transverse 'mini' laparotomy incision is made through the skin of the umbilical fossa. The skin edges are retracted with self-retaining retractors and the wound is deepened, incising and suture tagging the linea alba. The fascia overlying the peritoneum is cleared and the exposed peritoneum is incised vertically over a distance of 1 cm and suture tagged on each edge. (See Hasson, H.M. (1971) A modified instrument and method for laparoscopy. *American Journal of Obstetrics and Gynecology* **110**(6), 886–887.)

Improving the laparoscopic view
M.J. Coptcoat

During a long and difficult laparoscopic procedure there is often a thin film of blood that in itself is not dangerous but causes widespread absorption of the white light used. The image seen on the monitor gradually becomes darker and darker. Aspiration of this blood is often very difficult and can never be complete.

One trick that not only helps to remove any clot but also improves the light intensity available is to introduce a white swab. This must not become too soaked in blood and sometimes a second clean swab is required. The fresh white swab should be placed in the background so that it reflects the maximum amount of light and the overall image will become startlingly more clear.

Laparoscopic suturing
M.J. Coptcoat

A continuous suture requires a knot at the beginning and at the end. This can be difficult and tedious for the inexperienced laparoscopic surgeon, but can be avoided with the simple technique of using an endoclip both at the beginning and on completion of the continuous suture (Fig. 19).

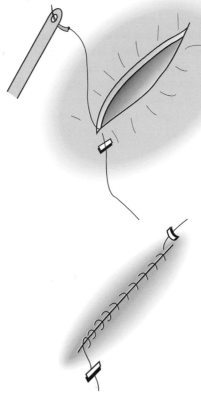

Figure 19

Endoscopic equipment tips

Resectoscope care
P.J.R. Boyd

Here is a manoeuvre I have recently started to use with all endoscopic resections. I use a Storz resectoscope, but others may also be suitable.

The object is to make sure that the resecting loop fits correctly into the sheath before starting to resect. The stimulus came from a number of sheaths damaged by trainees.

With the sheath in the bladder and the working piece ready to resect, I loosen the 30° scope and withdraw it while keeping the loop in view. The telescope only needs to be pulled back 1 cm or less to see the position of the loop in relation to the cutting edge of the sheath (Fig. 20). It is surprising how often minor adjustments are needed.

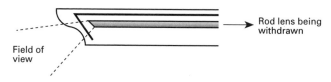

Rod lens being withdrawn

Field of view

Figure 20

To clean diathermy loops, leads and points
D.G. Arkell

The end of a diathermy loop or point that has become charred with blood clot, tumour and debris can be easily cleaned by using a small piece of nylon pan scourer. The scourer, available from most supermarkets or hardware stores, can be cut into 7.5 x 5 cm pieces and sterilized, then either packed separately or incorporated into the cystoscope, resectoscope or open surgical packs.

Preventing thermal injury to drapes or the patient when using an unprotected light cable
P.J. O'Boyle

Using a microvideo operating system requires a high light intensity to ensure good picture definition. Many light cables are now manufactured with a recess which prevents the extremely hot fibre bundles from coming into contact with the patient and drapes. Just as many, however, do not have this feature and a carelessly placed fibre-optic transmission cable can readily cause drapes to smoulder and even result in a patient burn.

A very simple tip is to keep a kidney dish on the patient's abdomen and always put the light source in the kidney dish when unconnected. The most vulnerable times are during the initial setting up process and at the end of the operation.

How to ensure good colour balance during microvideo operating procedures
P.J. O'Boyle

It can be very frustrating when demonstrating the benefits of microvideo operating to find that there is an excessively red picture despite repeatedly using the white colour balance and adjusting the red filters on the video camera. This is even before you start operating. It is commonly assumed that the video camera is not functioning properly, but it is actually very rare for solid state cameras to malfunction providing the connecting lead is in good repair. The reason for the excessively red picture is that someone has been fiddling with the television monitor. Adjusting the chromatic balance on the monitor effectively white-balances the telescope allowing you to obtain a perfect picture.

Open
Urology

General points

Prepping the patient is fun . . . if you know how!
P.J. O'Boyle

It is amazing how often patients arrive in the operating theatre unprepared. In particular, the suprapubic prep is omitted and can cause irritation on a busy list. One of the many little jewels shown to me by Richard Turner-Warwick makes the task simple, effective and easy to demonstrate to others.

A 50 : 50 mix of Savlon and Hibitane is generously applied over the suprapubic area. A sharp safety razor is used to remove unwanted hair while the skin is kept under firm tension. The trick is to gently move the razor backwards and forwards *but never to lift it from the skin*. All the hair is rapidly, easily and completely removed without resorting to further washing or the use of Elastoplast strapping.

Towelling up
R.D.C. Southcott

When putting on side towels for abdominal surgery fold the corners across towards the far side. They will then be less likely to fall on the floor while awaiting the other towels. Put the side towels on first and the larger top and bottom ones on afterwards to avoid any recesses under which swabs or instruments may hide.

If towelling up in the cystoscopy position, tuck the corner of the towel under the patient; it is easier and gives a wide diagonal spread of towels below.

Skirting the umbilicus

C.G. Fowler

When making a midline incision grasp the skin fold on one side of the umbilicus in tissue-holding forceps like an Allis. Pull the skin across the midline towards the other side of the patient. Make a straight midline incision. Hey presto! When you release the tension in the skin you will find it has skirted the umbilicus (Fig. 21).

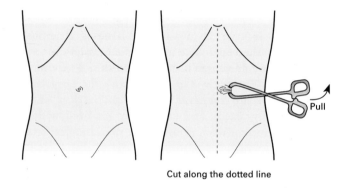

Cut along the dotted line

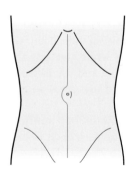

Figure 21

The Bristol roll
J. McLoughlin

This particular trick of packing abdominal contents has been shown to many Bristol trainees by Roger Feneley (who was originally shown it by Reg Lawrie). It overcomes the problem of the bowels tending to fall into the abdominal/pelvic wound despite careful initial packing off with wet swabs.

The technique involves placing wet packs under retractor blades as usual. A small green surgical drape is then soaked and wrung until moist. This is then loosely folded over and over again prior to placement at the bottom of the wound (i.e. beneath the initial wet swabs). Its shape assumes a U shape with either end pointing down into the pelvis, the middle being placed upwards.

Bits of plastic
R.G. Willis

David Thomas of Leeds introduced me to Vygon infant feeding tubes (6 F and 8 F, 125 cm long, ref 391.06 and 391.08). They have a multitude of uses because they are very long, have a syringe connector and possess radiological markers. I use them as ureteric stents in ileal conduits for testing ureteric patency (unlike ureteric catheters you can aspirate with a syringe and ensure the tip is in the bladder).

They are also valuable as short-term stents following open ureteric surgery where they can be passed down into the bladder, checked by aspiration, cut to length and their upper end threaded into the kidney. They usually stay put while the bladder is catheterized but, following catheter removal, about 50% of patients will pass them spontaneously saving their formal removal later (this particular point was cribbed from Philip Powell of Newcastle).

Lastly, they make a good short-term ureteric stent following re-implantation of the ureter, at which time they can be passed up along the ureter and their lower end brought out through the bladder and abdominal wall to drain into a bile bag. By cutting the securing stitch they are easily pulled out after 8–10 days (cribbed from David Thomas of Leeds).

Securing a tube drain
C.G. Fowler

If you are going to leave a drain it makes sense to fix it so that it will not fall out. Most people seem to secure a tube drain by multiple loops with a single throw on either side. This gives an effect like Malvolio's cross garters: the loops fall down and loosen. There is a better method.

Make a clove hitch from two loops of thread and pass them over the tube (Fig. 22). These loops can be tightened accurately onto the tube by the first throw of a reef knot. The second throw secures the knot. Tie another reef knot a short distance away so that the drain has a sort of mesentery brought out. The drain stitch can then be sutured to the skin. Because the suture can be snugged firmly to the tube, it will not slip.

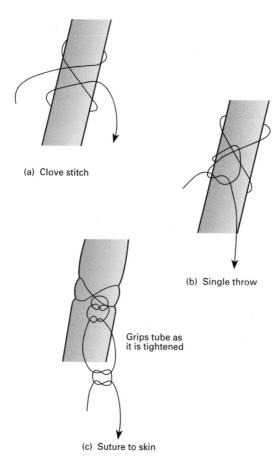

(a) Clove stitch

(b) Single throw

Grips tube as
it is tightened

(c) Suture to skin

Figure 22

Making the best of a short suture length in a deep dark hole
J. McLoughlin

When working deep in the pelvis or abdomen you will occasionally complete a suture line with only a short length remaining, which you need to use to throw your knot. While you can struggle to tie the knot with what is usually a short loop of suture, a simpler solution is to slip a length of any available suture material (e.g. vicryl) through the loop using a pair of right-angled forceps (Fig. 23). This in effect provides an extension to your suture allowing you to throw the knot and it can be pulled out before cutting the ends to length. It takes only a few seconds but can save a lot of aggravation. This was shown to me by Gary Lieskovsky of Los Angeles.

Koontz closure for re-closing a ruptured Pfannenstiel incision
J. McLoughlin

There are occasions where you need to re-close a burst incision in the early post-operative period. Re-suturing a Pfannenstiel incision, e.g. following complex pelvic surgery, can be very difficult as the rectus sheaths become embedded in a mush of oedematous angry tissue. In addition, these patients are often frail and may have been opened using the same incision previously. I was taught a closure technique based on a modification of that described by Koontz that is both simple and reliable.

Once you have made sure there is no adherent small bowel on the underbelly of the rectus muscle or adjacent peritoneum, appose the rectus muscles using a combination of horizontal and vertical interrupted mattress sutures with a 742 prolene or other non-absorbable suture.

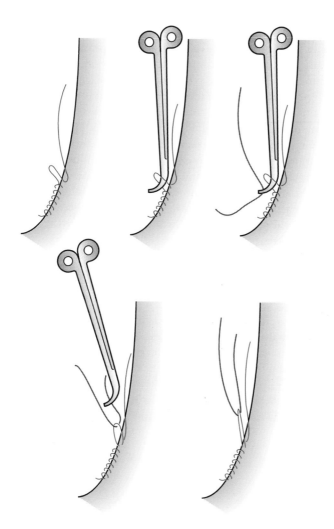

Figure 23

The next step is to close the rectus sheath. If you simply suture the tissue in the area of mush where you imagine the sheath to lie you will be left with a rather weak, uncertain closure. Instead, pass the prolene through the superior skin flap to one side of the midline (going from out to in), a good 3–4 cm away from the wound edge. This suture passes down through and out of the superior sheath up into the inferior sheath, loops back into the superior rectus sheath and again out via the inferior sheath, exiting through the inferior aspect of the wound. The needle is then brought back through the wound edges as if you were using a horizontal mattress suture (Fig. 24). Repeat two or three times on either side of the midline. Do not tie these sutures at this stage but rather clip both ends.

These sutures are then elevated by pulling up on the clips, thus tenting up the rectus sheath enabling you to get a surprisingly good purchase of the rectus sheath and muscle, and allowing placement of a line of interrupted prolene sutures. These are tied as you go along.

The initial sutures are then tied. In doing so, the skin edges oppose and you have also effectively placed a series of deep tension sutures. These look a little unsightly but should remain *in situ* for at least 2 weeks before being removed, allowing time for the sutures that oppose the rectus sheath to heal without tension.

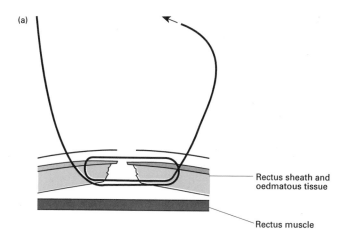

Rectus sheath and oedmatous tissue

Rectus muscle

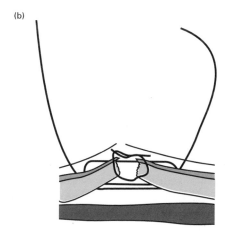

Sagittal view of the rectus sheath and muscle

Figure 24

Accurate diathermy haemostasis
A. Walsh

Good haemostasis and gentle tissue handling are essential to the craft of surgery. Some surgeons like to use ligatures while others prefer diathermy. One of the problems of using diathermy is that, whether a bleeding vessel is grasped by a haemostat or diathermy forceps, the tissue around the vessel is often caught as well, with the result that there is far more tissue coagulated than necessary. Every extra quantum of dead tissue in a wound gives an extra quantum of morbidity and encourages wound infection. Many years ago I learnt from the late T.J.D. Lane a technique that ensures that only the offending vessel is taken, a technique that appealed to my inherent laziness.

Let your assistant have the diathermy control pedal and the diathermy pencil, forceps, scissors or whatever. If right handed, you pick up the offending vessel with a fine non-toothed forceps held in your left hand. The assistant touches this vessel with the diathermy pencil and activates the current. You have full control of the proceedings because you can at any moment let go of the vessel. Non-toothed Adson forceps are excellent for this purpose. Manoeuvring is much easier if you have large toothed forceps, such as Bonney forceps, in your right hand and use this to hold nearby tissue to display the bleeding vessel. Even the most inexperienced assistant soon learns that when something is held in your left hand with non-toothed forceps it is to be touched with the diathermy probe.

This is an easy and quick technique. In a very large incision such as that for a radical nephrectomy, your assistant can control the bleeding in half the wound by keeping a hand lightly pressing on a swab occupying that half while you seal the vessels in the other half of the wound.

Renal

The cheese wire technique for partial nephrectomy
J.C. Smith

Professor Willard Goodwin of Los Angeles taught me a useful method of amputating part of the kidney.

The line of amputation is defined and if there is an obvious vessel supplying the pole it is ligated and the area of ischaemia visualized. The renal capsule is incised circumferentially and peeled back for 1 cm (Fig. 25b). A strong ligature (number 1 dexon) is placed round the kidney with a double throw on the knot (Fig. 25c). The pole is then ampu-

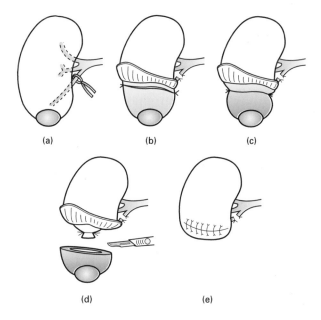

(a) (b) (c)

(d) (e)

Figure 25

tated by steadily tightening the ligature. The main renal artery may be occluded with a bulldog clip during the manoeuvre. The ligature is tightly tied and the pole amputated with a knife 0.5 cm distal to the ligature (Fig. 25d). Further haemostasis is obtained with 3/0 transfixion ligatures tied gently. If sufficient, the capsule may be sutured over the pole of the kidney.

Nephrectomy
A.B. Richards

In a difficult right nephrectomy for a large tumour, if operating through an anterior approach as I usually do, it can be extremely useful to tie the right renal artery between the cava and aorta at an early stage in the procedure (Fig. 26).

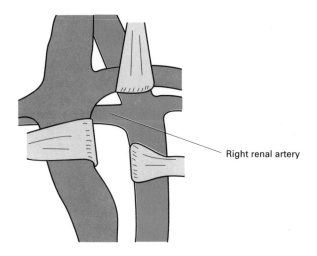

Right renal artery

Figure 26

Control of heavy intrarenal bleeding during stone surgery
A.R. de Bolla

Heavy intrarenal bleeding from the area of the calyceal neck is an occasional, but serious, problem during open and percutaneaous renal surgery. It is particularly dangerous in the case of a single kidney. The control of such a haemorrhage may be achieved by tightly packing the involved calyx, or indeed the whole renal pelvis, with 1 inch ribbon gauze. The ribbon is brought out to the surface via a separate nephrostomy. The patient is kept on antibiotics and the packing gently removed under anaesthetic 24–36 h later, usually without further mishap.

Though I have not personally used this technique to arrest haemorrhage after percutaneous surgery, it should be possible to introduce a ribbon down an Amplatz sheath if necessary.

Nephrectomy for the difficult kidney
M.A. Jones

Nephrectomy for the grossly infected kidney, xanthogranulomatous pyelonephritis and following drainage of a perinephric abscess can be a very hazardous operation. The major problems encountered can be adherence of inflammatory tissue to the colon or duodenum and inflammatory masses wrapped around the inferior vena cava. Nephrectomy through the loin is usually recommended, and in cases of difficulty a subcapsular nephrectomy is usually advised. In the presence of gross fibrosis or active inflammation it can be possible to find the wrong plane into the kidney via the loin approach and inadvertent damage to the bowel or the cava is not uncommon. My experience with such cases has led me to believe that the loin approach is unsatisfactory and that transabdominal nephrectomy is infinitely preferable.

The patient is positioned supine on the table with a small sandbag under the appropriate loin. A midline or supra-umbilical horizontal incision is used depending on the build of the patient. The colon, duodenum or duodeno-jejunal flexure are dissected from the perinephric mass as for a radical nephrectomy. Since the bowel is being mobilized from the kidney, damage is much less likely and where it occurs it is easily identified and repaired. The renal vessels are approached as for a radical nephrectomy and ligated in continuity. If the inflammatory mass is found to be involving the vena cava, the cava can be controlled with a Satinski clamp, if necessary and part of the caval side wall can be resected and the cava repaired with a vascular suture. Having secured control of the renal pedicle the kidney and perinephric mass are removed *en bloc* as for a radical nephrectomy. The renal bed is drained if gross sepsis is present and the abdomen is closed in the usual manner.

Since adopting this technique, I have found it to be a far safer and less hair-raising way of attempting nephrectomy in these circumstances, and of particular advantage in giving excellent access to the bowel and the main vasculature.

Securing the vascular pedicle during the difficult nephrectomy
M.J. Speakman

During radical nephrectomy it is accepted that, whenever possible, the renal artery should be ligated before the renal vein to avoid venous congestion. If this is difficult, however, a good tip is to place three 2/0 vicryl ligatures as in Fig. 27. Two of these pass around the renal vein alone, while the third, placed centrally, passes around both the renal artery and vein together. The two outer ligatures are then tied and the renal vein is divided between these two ligatures. The central ligature which is effectively now around only the renal artery itself is then ligated through the line of division of the renal vein. Thereby, arterial input is occluded and further appropriate dissection can proceed.

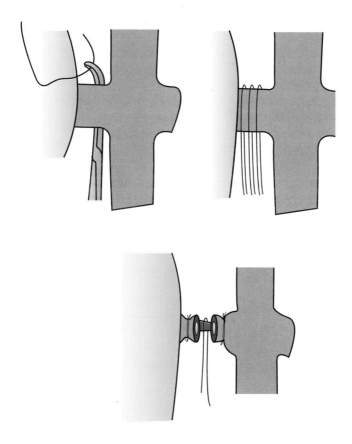

Figure 27

Nephrectomy
P.H. Smith

At nephrectomy the renal artery, renal vein and ureter have a disconcerting habit of retreating from the surgeon at the most vital moments. Bleeding from the two vessels is probably best prevented by double proximal ligation; the proximal ligatures being cut before the vessels are transected. The ureter, if mobilized to the pelvic brim (desirable lest a subsequent intervention be required to remove it), is difficult to ligate securely at this level. If the ligature is tied and cut before division, one never ends up with an oozing distal ureter deep in the pelvis.

Nephro-ureterectomy
G.B. Williams

Nephro-ureterectomy can nowadays be performed through a flank incision, as pre-operative staging can show if there is any extrarenal spread of urothelial disease. The ureter can be 'plucked' up from the bladder as it tents up behind the superior vesical artery.

At the check cystoscopy 3 months later, a double catheterizing slide should be used. Pass a 5 F ureteric catheter up the nephrectomized ureteric orifice via the catheterizing channel, and a bee-sting diathermy up the other. The intramural course of the nephrectomized ureter can be sliced open by the bee-sting electrode for the length of the intravesical ureter and the whole area fulgurated with an 8 F Otis electrode.

Through and through nephrostomy tube
G.C. Tresidder

The following notes will make the management — securing and changing — of nephrostomy tubes easier and more straightforward. This note should be read as an addendum to Tresidder (1957).

Once both ends of the nephrostomy tube have been brought out through the renal substance and skin, each is secured to the skin in the following way. A circumferential nylon suture should be tightened so that it indents the wall of the tube, thus constricting it slightly. After tying a second reef knot (see Securing a tube drain, pp. 54–55) next to the first one the suture is stitched to the immediately adjacent skin (Fig. 28).

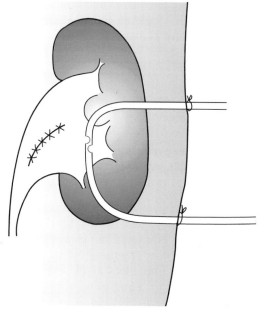

Figure 28

To change a nephrostomy tube, both the skin stitches are removed. The end emerging from the middle calyx is drawn out 1 cm and divided at skin level. A long plain nylon suture is passed through it, taking a bite 5 mm from the end of the new tube. The suture is tied so that the knot lies within the lumen of the tube. In a similar way two other sutures are placed equidistant from the first one and also from each other. The limb of the old tube emerging from the lower calyx is then drawn out and the rest of the old tube along with the new tube and three nylon sutures follow.

Next, it is established that the two openings in the nephrostomy tube lie within the ureteric pelvis. Then the nylon sutures are cut through and removed with the old tube. By laying the old tube alongside the new one it can be seen where the circumferential nylon sutures should be tied around the new tube. Applying surface spray and subcutaneous injection analgesia around the emerging nephrostomy tube, the nylon sutures are secured to the adjacent skin.

Reference
Tresidder, G.C. (1957) Nephrostomy. *British Journal of Urology*
   29, 130.

Stay sutures in the performance of an Anderson–Hynes pyeloplasty
D.W.W. Newling

One of the major problems that can be encountered in the performance of an Anderson–Hynes pyeloplasty is the twisting of the ureter before the final anastomosis is made. This can be prevented by inserting, before dismembering the pelvi–ureteric junction, two sutures in the upper ureter approximately 3 cm apart. With one suture it is possible for the ureter to turn through 180° and to be anastomosed to the pelvis, even with a stent in place, without the operator being aware that this has occurred. Two sutures, 3 cm apart, can prevent this happening.

Pyeloplasty and open ureterolithotomy
R.G. Notley

Put a small coin on the umbilicus when doing a retrograde ureterogram prior to pyeloplasty (Fig. 29). You can then relate the umbilicus to the pelvi–ureteric junction and make your anterior approach exactly over the junction. Using the coin in the umbilicus also used to be a good way of aiming your incision accurately when taking a check X-ray on the table prior to open ureterolithotomy. This is now a pretty rare operation.

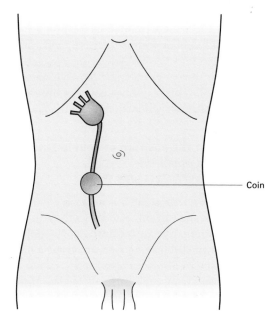

———— Coin

Figure 29

Ureter

A means of facilitating a psoas hitch during ureteric re-implantation
K.N. Bullock

During a Leadbetter–Politano ureteric re-implantation it may be necessary, if the bladder is opened vertically in the midline, to mobilize the contralateral side of the bladder to provide sufficient bladder mobility to permit re-implantation of the ureter and insertion of a psoas hitch without tension.

If the bladder is opened obliquely and then sutured in the opposite direction (like a pyloroplasty) sufficient oblique lengthening of the bladder is obtained to allow re-implantation and psoas hitching without tension, and without the need to mobilize the opposite side of the bladder by dividing the superior vesical vessels and the obliterated umbilical artery (Fig. 30). This shortens operating time and avoids problems with bleeding when mobilizing the bladder wall.

Confirmation of the position of double J stent inserted at open operation
J.C. Gingell

When placing a ureteric stent it is necessary to ensure that the distal end is sited in the bladder and not in the lower ureter. As an alternative to confirmation by either cystoscopy or radiological screening you can do so by incorporating a few extra steps into your operation.

Catheterize and empty the patient's bladder before he or she is turned to the lateral position. Fill the bladder with 150–200 ml of a solution of 1% methylene blue in 500 ml normal saline and spigot the catheter. Peform the operation

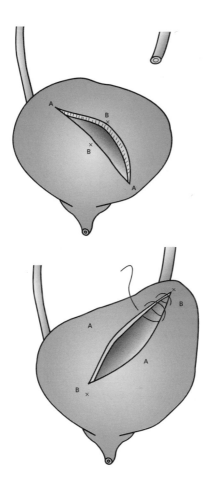

Figure 30

and insert the double J stent antegradely. As soon as the guide wire is removed, methylene blue effluxes from the side holes of the stent, confirming that it is placed within the bladder (Fig. 31). If the dye does not efflux directly, press gently on the suprapubic area. If the dye still does not

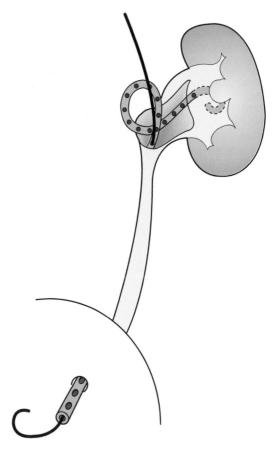

Figure 31

appear, the stent is not in the bladder and insertion must be attempted again.

As soon as you are happy, the urethral catheter should be unclamped and connected to closed drainage. The position of the stent can be confirmed by a standard X-ray in the post-operative period.

Finding the transected ureter
D.E. Sturdy

Urinary leakage from the incision after abdominal and pelvic surgery is a dramatic and potentially serious complication. Most ureteric injuries happen during operative procedures in the pelvis and involve the terminal 4–5 cm of the ureter.

A 40-year-old woman of short stature underwent an abdominal hysterectomy for uterine fibroids. A preliminary intravenous urogram (IVU) had demonstrated lateral and anterior displacement of the ureter within the pelvis. On the third post-operative day the wound, which was a low bikini-friendly incision, began to 'leak'. After 10 days a urological opinion was requested. The gynaecological operation note described 'heavy peroperative bleeding from the left uterine artery'. A repeat IVU revealed 'left-sided hydronephrosis and 'pooling' of dye in the left side of the pelvis. The left ureter is not adequately demonstrated.' Cystoscopy revealed a normal bladder and ureteric orifices, but a ureteric catheter could not be advanced for more than 2 cm up the left ureter and retrograde ureterography was unsuccessful. This investigation seemed to confirm damage to the left ureter at a low level near the bladder. The pelvis was re-explored through the previous Pfannenstiel incision. The divided distal ureter was found at the side of the bladder, foreshortened and coiled, while the tip of the retrograde catheter could be palpated, held up in one of the concertina loops (Fig. 32a). Gentle mobilization allowed 8 cm of viable ureter to be straightened. The next hour was spent in a vain attempt to find the proximal ureter; the exploration considerably hampered by poor access through the low transverse incision. A long left paramedian incision was performed and the proximal ureter found, convoluted like a spring, at L3 level, 3 cm below the renal pelvis (Fig. 32b). It was then a simple matter to straighten the ureter, and the gap between the two ends, which at first seemed unbridgeable, was easily closed by an anastomosis over a retrograde ureteric splint. The patient made an uneventful recovery.

There are lessons that can be learned here. Poking about in the pelvis through inadequate access is both unrewarding and inadvisable. Despite all indicators pointing towards a 'low' ureteric injury, this was not the case. The muscularity of the ureter (90% muscle), stretched like a bow string over the fibroid enlargement, had produced a coiled spring-like effect and wide retraction of the transected ends.

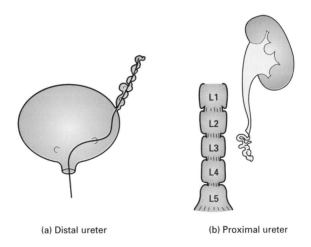

(a) Distal ureter   (b) Proximal ureter

Figure 32

There are also conclusions that can be drawn. For reasons of inadequate access, cosmesis should have been a secondary consideration both at the time of the original hysterectomy and the subsequent intervention to repair the damaged ureter. A salvage operation for repair of a transected ureter demands adequate exposure of the entire length of the intra-abdominal and pelvic ureter. The salvage operator must not assume that the ureter has been injured at the site nominated by the referring surgeon nor, in this case, necessarily at the site suggested by pre-operative investigations.

Lowering the right renal vein
G. Williams

Strictures of the upper right ureter as a result of stones, trauma or tuberculosis are often difficult to deal with via an end-to-end anastomosis due to lack of ureteric length. Up to 5–7.5 cm of extra length can be obtained by lowering the right renal vein.

The right kidney is fully mobilized and the renal artery and vein stripped of all adventitia. The vena cava is cleared for about 7.5 cm below the insertion of the right renal vein. The renal artery is clamped with a soft vascular clamp and a Satinski clamp is placed on the vena cava at the insertion of the renal vein. The renal vein is divided and the venotomy in the vena cava closed with a two-layer continuous running 6/0 prolene suture.

The kidney can now be brought 5–7.5 cm inferiorly. The Satinski clamp is now placed on the vena cava at this point and incised. Using two double-ended 6/0 prolene sutures, the renal vein is re-anastomosed to the vena cava and finally the clamp is removed from the renal artery.

Exposure of the termination of an ectopic ureter or other anomalies in the posterior urethra

J.H. Johnston

When upper hemi nephro-ureterectomy is required for the treatment of an ectopic supernumerary ureter draining into the posterior urethra, the ureter need ordinarily be mobilized and excised only within the limits of the abdominal incision. However, on occasion the resulting ureteric stump may cause further problems such as persisting infection or calculus formation. In such circumstances its removal is required; the preferred approach is transvesical.

Through a suprapubic abdominal incision, the anterior wall of the bladder is opened in routine fashion and a self-retaining retractor is inserted. The trigone and posterior wall are divided (Fig. 33a) exposing the ureteric stump (Fig. 33b) which can then be traced to its insertion either into the urethra or into an often cystically dilated seminal vesicle. In either circumstance, complete excision of the intra-urethral structure is required. The vasa deferentia can be recognized and, if not too adherent, can be preserved.

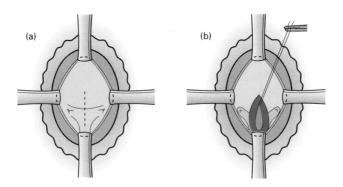

Figure 33

The same approach is useful for diverticulectomy in boys with a posterior urethral diverticulum often, coincidentally, associated with hypospadias where the diverticulum is causing urinary infection associated with recurrent epididymitis. In such a case, the vasa often open into the diverticulum so that removal inevitably leads to bilateral vasectomy. The surgeon may console him- or herself with the thought that the boy who has had bilateral epididymitis is likely to be rendered infertile in any event.

This transtrigonal transvesical technique has been employed by myself in the older prepubertal child. Whether it works for adults I do not know for the good reason that I have never had the opportunity to try it. No doubt someone will let me know.

Exposure of the pelvic ureter with a small incision
A. Walsh

This is a neat and simple way of exposing the ureter at the pelvic brim, as for an appendicectomy, but which remains extraperitoneal. After going through the transversalis fascia you put a large swab into the wound, press it very firmly medially with the thumb and then replace your thumb, so to speak, with a self-retaining retractor such as a Deaver, which is opened up as widely as possible pushing the swab medially. There, to your great surprise the first time you do it, is the ureter easily visible at the bottom of the wound.

Bladder

Cystectomy
R.G. Willis

The principal difficulty with this operation is the lack of room to manoeuvre as one works one's way down each side of the bladder (especially in men) securing the blood supply. It is often difficult or impossible to place two angled clamps on these vessels due to the confined space. Attempts to ligate in continuity result in both ligatures lying so close together that it is impossible to cut between them.

My tip is to use a combination of these two methods. First, pinching the tissues between your finger and thumb helps define a suitable window between leashes of vesical vessels so that an angled clamp can be passed through the 'mesentery'. Second, having defined the bladder end of the pedicle, ligate in continuity so that this tie (inevitable anyway) lies on the bladder end of the pedicle. Leave the tie uncut, use it to stretch the pedicle gently towards the bladder and slide an angled clamp *down* the pedicle towards the pelvic side wall before applying it (Fig. 34). In this way the pedicle is securely clamped with only one piece of metal work in the area, and comfortably away from the first tie so that the pedicle can be divided and ligated safely. And so on to the next deeper set of vesical vessels!

Ligation of the ureters during cystectomy, prior to urinary diversion
D.W.W. Newling

When cystectomy and urinary diversion into a conduit or continent reservoir is to be carried out, I have found it extremely useful to tie the ureters at the same time as the

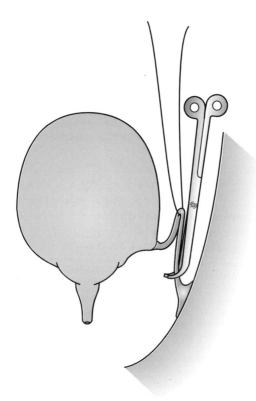

Figure 34

internal iliac arteries are controlled, prior to cystectomy. This results in dilatation of the ureters making for an easy uretero–intestinal anastomosis at the end of the procedure. I have never come across any temporary or permanent evidence of deterioration in renal function as a result of this manoeuvre and have invariably found that the subsequent uretero–ileal or ureterocolonic anastomosis is relatively easy to perform.

The retro-ureteric plane for cystectomy

J. McLoughlin

This manoeuvre is used by Gary Sibley at the Bristol Royal Infirmary. It allows for a relatively bloodless dissection along the plane that exists behind and around the ureter, bringing the operator onto the lateral vesical pedicle early on, and affords good access for placement of a clip prior to division of the pedicle. It is especially useful in the male pelvis.

The ureter is mobilized and pulled forwards. Then, the index finger is placed down behind (Fig. 35). This plane is opened up by gentle dissection with MacIndoes scissors using an opening movement rather than a closing (cutting) motion. Once begun, this plane can be developed with the index finger. The pedicles can be palpated laterally (as a band-like structure), and can be taken in a series of bites using either Roberts or similar forceps.

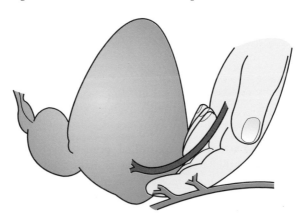

Figure 35

Cystectomy
C.A.C. Charlton

During cystectomy, when mobilizing the ureters at the level of division of the common iliac artery, isolate the proximal 1 cm of the internal iliac artery and ligate it in continuity. This limits bleeding at later stages of cystectomy. Do not do this if the inferior mesenteric artery has been ligated from large bowel surgery as severe ischaemia of the rectum may result.

When constructing an ileal conduit, particularly if more than 1 year has elapsed following radiotherapy, the integrity and safety of the uretero–ileal anastomosis is protected by the use of two 12 inch uretero–ileal stents. Each one is secured by using 4/0 catgut with a cutting needle through both the ureteric wall and the stent, which is loosely tied. These stitches dissolve at 10 days and are withdrawn by gentle traction as they emerge from the ileal spout.

Cystectomy
R.D.C. Southcott

Tie off the internal iliac arteries in continuity at the beginning of a cystectomy, *but* be sure to use thick thread to avoid cutting through the vessels.

Cystectomy
G.B. Williams

Total radical cystectomy is often complicated by torrential venous bleeding from the inferior vesical veins. This occurs when the vesical venous drainage is inadvertently transected; the venous effluent from the leg and inferior vena cava vanishes up the sucker. Time spent finding the internal iliac vein (usually behind the internal iliac artery) is rewarding. It can be ligated in continuity — before that inadvertent transection of the venous effluent of the bladder occurs. It is well worthwhile seeing the procedure under direct vision, rather than under the surface of rising blood.

Cystectomy — ligation of the vesical pedicles
J. Vinnicombe

Identification and ligation of vascular components of the vesical pedicles can often be difficult, and division and ligation may become a haemorrhagic procedure.

A tip learned from my late chief at St Thomas's has proved invaluable over the years: use a Millin's boomerang needle with the needle tip blunted. This will penetrate the pedicle tissue without damage to the vessels and can be applied initially close to the pelvic wall and subsequently close to the bladder, leaving a safe plane for division of the pedicle between ligatures. I normally use this technique two or three times on each side of the bladder.

Split cuff ileal stomas
R.G. Notley

The cuffed ileal conduit spout, with full-thickness eversion and primary mucocutaneous suture, both reduces the risk of stenosis and facilitates collection of urine. Eversion of the spout is made easier and the spout bulk reduced by the 'split cuff technique'.

The ileum is delivered through a cored incision onto the abdominal wall and is anchored with a few intraperitoneal sutures. The main abdominal wound is closed. The spout of the ileum is then steadied by placing a finger in its lumen and the seromuscular layer of the distal half is incised longitudinally down to, but not through, the mucosa at two or three equidistant points around its circumference

(Fig. 36). These myotomies relax the distal half of the spout. A tissue forceps is passed into the lumen to grasp the proximal mucosa, and the distal part of the ileum can then be everted simply to form the final cuffed spout that is secured to the skin edges with interrupted catgut sutures.

In the immediate post-operative period the appearance of the stoma may appear somewhat alarming as, at the outer

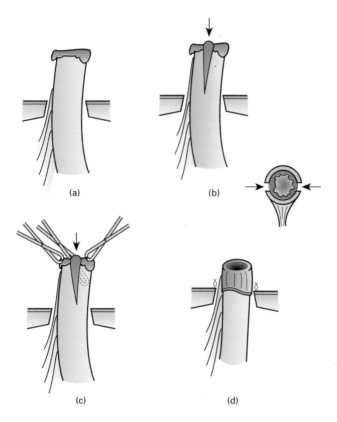

(a)

(b)

(c)

(d)

Figure 36

layer of the cuff, everted mucosa becomes congested, purple and oedematous owing to the initial ischaemia consequent on the longitudinal myotomies in the everted portion. By 4–6 weeks the mucosa recovers its colour and consistency, the swelling subsides and this, together with the atrophy of the everted muscle layers, reduces the bulk of the spout, making placement of the appliance and its concealment easier.

How to tension the sutures in a Burch colposuspension

P.J. O'Boyle

Adjusting the tension of the sutures is the key to success in any colposuspension. Frequently, after placing the suspending sutures through the iliopectineal line, it is technically awkward to maintain the desired tension while tying the knot. A useful tip, which I may have picked up from a sailing friend, is to take the equivalent of a 'round turn' on the iliopectineal suture by passing the needle through the line twice. This gives a fixed point for one end of the suture and allows the tension to be adjusted easily and locked by a series of half hitches.

An aid to vaginal surgery of vesicovaginal fistulas

A. Walsh

Many simple vesicovaginal fistulas are easy to close with the patient lying downward in the Sims' position and the posterior vaginal wall elevated with the Sims' retractor, designed specifically for this purpose. The corrugation of the vaginal mucosa does, however, make it difficult to be certain that the fistula has been fully excised and that no mucosal bridge, however small, remains uniting the vaginal and bladder mucosas.

This difficulty is solved simply by passing a large Foley catheter from the vagina through the fistula into the bladder. The balloon is then inflated to perhaps 30 or 40 ml. Now, traction on the Foley catheter will bring the fistula into very clear view and make full excision easy.

Barium sedimentation and the detection of enterovesical fistulas
R.P. MacDonagh

Enterovesical fistulas are uncommon, accounting for approximately 1 : 3000 admissions to hospital. The diagnosis is essentially a clinical one, dependent upon eliciting the classic symptoms of pneumaturia and faecaluria, present in 67 and 45% of patients, respectively.

Traditionally, confirmation of the diagnosis rested upon a combination of cystoscopy and barium enema. At cystoscopy, however, a fistula is seen only in one-third of patients and a barium enema demonstrates the presence of an enterovesical communication in less than 40% of patients. An alternative investigation is computerized tomography, which although inaccurate in direct visualization of the fistula does identify air in the urinary bladder in up to 90% of patients with enterovesical fistulas.

The diagnostic accuracy of a barium enema can be significantly improved by collecting all urine passed by the patient for 24 h from the conclusion of the barium study. In the majority of patients with enterovesical fistulas, even those not visible radiologically, a white layer of barium can be seen to settle on the bottom of the 24-h container. In cases where the fistula is very small and the quantity of barium in the urine is insufficient to form a definitive layer, it is possible to X-ray the container and identify the barium as radio-opaque specks throughout the urine.

As a barium enema is invariably indicated in patients

with suspected enterovesical fistulas to elucidate any underlying colorectal pathology, this additional test is easy to perform, diagnostic and, when positive, prevents the need for any further additional investigation.

This top tip was told to me by W.T. Lawrence (Eastbourne) in 1991.

Prostate

The value of an urethral sound during retropubic prostatectomy
R.C.L. Feneley

The majority of urologists now enucleate the prostatic lobes during retropubic prostatectomy via an intra-urethral approach. Difficulty can be encountered entering the prostatic urethra, particularly if there is asymmetry of the gland. To facilitate this approach, a urethral sound can be passed through the urethra to localize the prostatic urethra.

This manoeuvre is used when the prostate has been exposed retropubically. Stay sutures are placed in the capsule of the prostate and a transverse incision made across the capsule (Fig. 37). At this point, the urethral sound (18 or 22 F) is passed into the bladder and gradually withdrawn and, by depressing the handle, the tip of the sound will come out through the transverse incision in the prostate, thus identifying the prostatic urethra. As the sound is withdrawn from the urethra, a pair of long scissors is passed into the prostatic urethra and opened. Digital examination of the prostatic urethra can then be performed and a bladder neck retractor placed *in situ*. Enucleation of the prostatic lobes can then proceed.

LATERAL VIEW

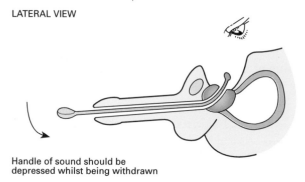

Handle of sound should be
depressed whilst being withdrawn

SUPERIOR VIEW

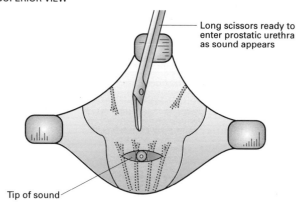

Long scissors ready to
enter prostatic urethra
as sound appears

Tip of sound

Figure 37

Retropubic prostatectomy
D.J. Oakland

When enucleating the prostate during a retropubic prostatectomy one's finger somtimes encounters several tough
strands at the apex of the gland. These may have to be cut
with scissors and it is helpful to know which 'strand' is the
urethra. A Foley catheter passed as far as the prostatic cavity makes it easy to decide which is the urethra. This can
then be cut across cleanly, avoiding accidental avulsion of
part of the membranous urethra. The same catheter is then
used for bladder drainage.

Post-prostatectomy perineal traction suture
to obliterate the prostatic cavity
P.J. O'Boyle

When a very large prostate has been enucleated, a considerable prostatic cavity is left which can give rise to troublesome
bleeding and may even require further exploration and packing. N.O.K. Gibbon devised a useful little manoeuvre that
rapidly and effectively obliterates the cavity.

A fine Stamey needle is passed from the perineum (as for
a perineal prostatic biopsy) and traverses the prostatic
cavity and bladder neck. A stout nylon suture is retrieved
from inside the bladder and brought out through the perineum. A further pass higher in the bladder neck collects
the other end of the suture and brings it out of the perineum
also. The process is repeated on the other side.

Tension can then be applied to the perineal sutures which
pull the bladder neck into the prostatic cavity, invaginating
and obliterating it. The sutures are then tied over two
dental rolls on each side of the urethra and the obliterated
cavity inspected once more before closing the capsule. The
sutures are removed at 48 h.

Freyer's fingers

N.O.K. Gibbon

My contribution concerns prostatectomy and I offer just three tips. Freyer's finger tips you could say!

1 *Freyer's finger dissection.* This points the way to the secret of his enormous success: complete removal of the adenomas. After referring to the high mortality from partial prostatectomy, he added '. . . in a very large proportion of cases the bladder failed to regain its power of expelling the urine. Furthermore, however good the initial result there was . . . no immunity against recurrent outgrowth or generalised enlargement of the gland . . .' (Freyer, 1906, p. 34). This argument applies equally well to the long-term results of other forms of adenectomy. Before Freyer's day, transurethral crushing and cautery had been tried and given up. Even nowadays, transurethral resection is commonly incomplete (sometimes grossly so — I could tell some horror stories to cap those of the 1930s (Lewis & Carroll, 1933)) and the lack of consistently good results still threatens to bring urology into disrepute. Moreover, a critical attitude is surely indicated towards the introduction of newer methods of prostatic destruction (heating, laser) which are likely to leave significant amounts of adenoma behind.

2 *Freyer's finger touch.* This enables the surgeon to assess the completeness of his or her operation. Referring to his new 'radical' procedure, Freyer stated 'After removal of the tumour, with a finger in the bladder and another in the rectum, I could feel that there was no prostatic substance left behind' (Freyer, 1901a). Elsewhere, he added '. . . the portion of the gland not involved in the tumour having been atrophied by pressure' (Freyer, 1901b). J.P. Blandy, in his textbook of urology (Blandy, 1976), used this strict criterion of a complete transurethral resection of the bladder, insisting that the bladder must be empty and the instrument out.

However, it should be added that with small adenomas a variable shell of normal gland may be felt post-operatively if atrophy has been incomplete. After adopting this rigorous policy in 1972 our long-term results improved noticeably.

3 *Freyer's finger pressure.* Freyer used blunt dissection to minimize bleeding during enucleations, which were carried out with the tip of his right (and occasionally left) index finger. The sharpest instrument used inside the bladder was his finger nail. He was not content with these precautions, however, and at the end of the operation applied pressure to the prostatic bed which was a logical and highly successful manoeuvre. He stated 'The contractility of the cavity will be greatly facilitated by pressing its opposing surface together by the points of the fingers in the bladder and in the rectum respectively' (Freyer, 1906, p. 44). Again, 'By thoroughly kneading the opposed surfaces together in this manner the contraction of the cavity and its diminution in size are facilitated and haemorrhage is thus arrested' (Freyer, 1906, p. 72). (Of course, after transurethral operations, counter pressure is provided by the pubic bones or by a hand over the lower abdomen.)

It was in the 1950s, while doing the profoundly taxing cold punch resections that I discovered the value of rectal finger pressure in rendering prominent the tissue to be removed and in reducing the calibre of blinding arterial bleeders. Over the years, the pressure technique has gradually included the management of all resections and enucleation. It proved particularly valuable during anaesthetic extubation and even back on the ward when bleeding recurred. It was not until many years later that I read Freyer's original papers in detail. Then I wished they had been compulsory reading for all surgical students! At least we might have been spared the illogicality of packing the prostatic cavity.

Postscript. Freyer reduced his mortality down to 3% towards the end of his first 1000 cases — without blood transfusions, antibiotics, modern anaesthesia or intensive care and without modern drainage equipment. Patients flocked from all over the world to be in his trustworthy hands. I do not know what his right index finger looked like after all those operations, but mine has big Heberden's nodes with ulnar deviation of the terminal phalanx (the left being fairly normal). This is a small price to pay for a complete job. Whatever procedure eventually replaces enucleation must be equally effective. At present, our long-term results are almost certainly much less satisfactory than his were.

References

Blandy, J.P. (ed.) (1976) *Urology*. Blackwell Scientific Publications.

Freyer, P.J. (1901a) Total extirpation of the prostate for radical cure of enlargement of that organ. *British Medical Journal* 20 July, 125–129.

Freyer, P.J. (1901b) Quoted by J.S. McLaren. *British Medical Journal* 17 August, 435.

Freyer, P.J. (1906) *Enlargement of the Prostate*, 3rd edn. Baillère, Tindall and Cox, London.

Lewis, B. and Carroll, G. (1933) Prostatic resection without the moonlight roses. *Urologic and Cutaneous Review* **37**, 1–7.

Radical prostatectomy

G.B. Williams

Ligation of the dorsalis penis venous complex is mandatory at the start of radical total prostatectomy. Sometimes, the dorsalis penis complex is deeper and thicker than you think and after confident ligation, proximal transection of the venous complex is complicated by torrential bleeding because you did not ligate all of it.

A large pack should be placed and pressure applied. A second incision, transversely across the root of the penis is made and the same procedure performed as for venous leakage in impotence. Ligate the dorsalis penis vein below the pubis — then go back above the pubis and take out the pack.

Reconstructive

Bloodless incision of the small bowel for a clam enterocystoplasty
M.H. Ashken

Following isolation of a length of ileum for use in a clam enterocystoplasty, the anti-mesenteric border needs incision throughout its length. To avoid any bleeding from the

(a)

(b)

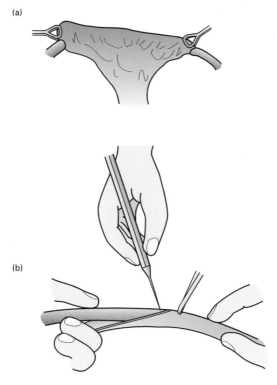

Figure 38

bowel wall it is a useful tip to pass a large silastic chest tube drain through the lumen of the isolated ileum (Fig. 38a, p. 93). The anti-mesenteric wall is then incised with a diathermy needle keeping the ileum tensely opposed to the silastic tube. This is then a bloodless procedure (Fig. 38b, p. 93) which is good for one's view and morale.

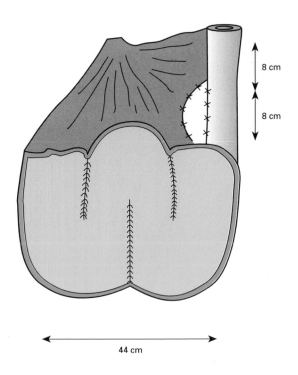

8 cm

8 cm

44 cm

Figure 39

Constructing a hemi-Kock ileocystoplasty
W.F. Hendry

In constructing a hemi-Kock ileocystoplasty it is important to get the proportions of detubularized bowel, which form the new bladder, to remaining tubularized bowel, which replaces the lower ureters, correctly balanced. It is also important to be sure to take enough bowel. The recommended dimensions are illustrated in Fig. 39 (*opposite*) and are based on those published in the *Journal of the Royal Society of Medicine*.

The simplest way to ensure that enough ileum is taken is to take a 60 cm length of ligature and lay it along the ileum. This is folded over on itself and folded over again to leave 15 cm, which should be the length of the unopened portion. This can then easily be marked off, and construction of the new bladder can proceed without further delay. I find a 2/0 chromic catgut and a straight needle holder allows the necessary suturing to be done with the minimum of delay.

Reference
Hendry, W.F., Christmas, T.J. and Shepherd, J.H. (1991) *Journal of the Royal Society of Medicine* **84**, 709–712.

Penis and scrotum

Bloodless day case surgery
D.G. Arkell

One way of ensuring that small open procedures (such as epididymal cyst excisions, hydrocoeles, etc.) present few post-operative problems is to use a neodymiumyttrium–aluminium–garnet (YAG) laser, set at low power (15–20 W) coupled with a contact sapphire probe to carry out all the incision work after the initial skin incision has been made. By dividing tissue under tension with such a probe a blood-less field results and post-operative healing is quick and painless. This method is particularly useful for excising anogenital condylomas and causes minimal scarring.

Local anaesthesia in circumcision
J. Cumming

Circumcision is usually performed under general anaesthesia supplemented with a penile block. I have found that the dorsal nerve block is insufficient for a complete block when the procedure is carried out under local anaesthetic alone.

There are nerves travelling along the urethra/spongiosum which supply the frenulum and ventral surface of the penis. A separate infiltration of lignocaine (1–2%) around the ventral surface of the spongiosum, near the tip of the penis, anaesthetizes this area effectively (Fig. 40).

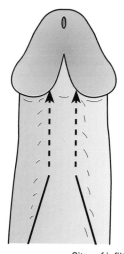

Sites of infiltration

Ventral surface

Figure 40

The tight frenulum and circumcision

J. Cumming

In such cases, the frenulum usually appears tight when the foreskin is retracted. When a circumcision is to be performed this can be released at the same time. It is usual to carry the skin incision distally towards the urethral meatus so that the extra length of shaft can be taken to the frenulum.

My tip is to incise the frenulum close to the glans and close the circumcision, leaving the frenular artery incision alone. The appearance is of an inverted Y-plasty (Fig. 41). Close the circumcision with 3/0 or 4/0 subcuticular absorbable suture taking care not to draw the suture tight.

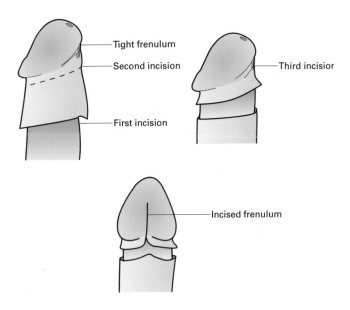

Figure 41

Catching the dreaded frenular artery at circumcision
R.H. Whitaker

The two layers (skin and mucosa) are incised so that the required amount of each remains but the mucosa is left attached by a 4 mm bridge at the frenular area. This bridge of mucosa, containing the frenular artery(ies), is stretched over a finger and the epithelial lining incised ever so carefully until the artery or arteries are exposed (Fig. 42). With the back of the knife blade the mucosa on each side of the bridge is pushed back and forth until there is enough room for a 5/0 catgut tie to be applied to the vessel(s). The rest of the procedure can be completed in the knowledge that severe post-operative bleeding from the frenular artery cannot occur.

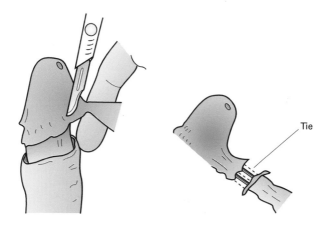

Tie

Figure 42

Correcting penile curvature
P.M.T. Weston

One of the disadvantages of Nesbitt's operation is the partial detumescence caused by incision and opening of the corpora cavernosa, making correction a matter of guesswork. This can be simply obviated by a point of technique

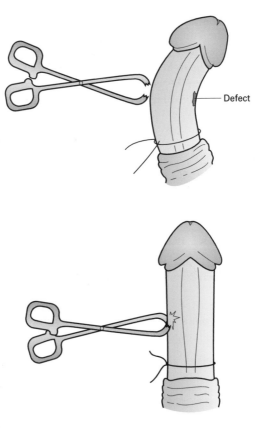

Defect

Figure 43

demonstrated to me during my training (R.W.M. Rees, personal communication). Allis tissue forceps are used to take bites of tunica opposite the site of maximum curvature until the deformity is corrected (Fig. 43). The forceps are left closed in position and enable excision of the correct amount of tunica to be subsequently effected. This technique also facilitates accurate corporeal plication.

An aid to Nesbitt's operation for Peyronie's disease
K.N. Bullock

During correction of erectile deformity, it can be difficult to assess how large should be the wedges of corpora excised to correct the deformity.

Following degloving of the penis, an artificial erection is induced using saline injection and a tourniquet around the base of the penis. Using Allis tissue forceps, the corpora can then be grasped directly opposite the bend to evert the tunica albuginea. The position of the forceps can be adjusted, squeezing the tunical tissue together, until the deformity is corrected.

Once the penis is straight, the forceps are removed and the tourniquet released. The Allis forceps leave an indentation in the surface of the tunica albuginea which marks where the elliptical incisions need to be made for the Nesbitt's procedure. Once the ellipses have been excised and the defects closed, a further artificial erection will confirm that the penis is straight, thereby removing the element of guesswork involved in how much tunica is excised.

A simple aid to correction of penile curvature
I.K. Dickinson

This manoeuvre allows the operator to both stabilize the penis and perform an artificial erection during procedures to correct penile curvature. Insert a stay suture into the glans penis and then insert a 19 G butterfly needle through the glans into the corpus cavernosum. Tie the stay suture around the butterfly wings. Apply the clip to the distal end of the stay suture (Fig. 44).

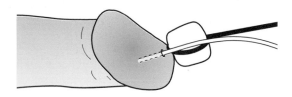

Figure 44

Simple vasectomy under local anaesthesia
R.J. Luck

Trap the vas between the thumb and first two fingers so that it is held against stretched scrotal skin. A 2 ml syringe containing 1% xylocaine attached to a 21 G needle is used to infiltrate the skin over the vas. Then, without withdrawing it completely, the needle is slipped under the vas (injecting as you go). The needle is pushed on until it emerges through the skin on the side of the vas away from the entry point, thus trapping the vas between the needle and the bridge of skin (Fig. 45). The needle should be so close to the vas that the skin over the vas is stretched.

The syringe is removed leaving the needle in position and

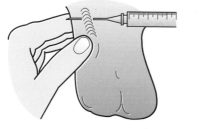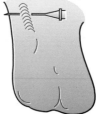

Figure 45

a 0.75 cm transverse incision is made in the scrotal skin into, but not cutting, the vas. Using sharp-pointed strabismus scissors, the adventitia is separated from the vas by opening and closing the points either side of the vas. The scissors are then passed under the vas which can be lifted with the scissors into the wound and grasped with Dunhill artery forceps.

The needle is removed and the vas can be delivered out of the scrotum. A length of vas is then excised and tied back 'hockey stick' fashion. The cut vas is returned to the scrotum. No skin stitch is required and the scrotal incision is covered by a dry dressing held in place with tight underpants. The operation of bilateral vasectomy takes about 15 min.

Vasectomy and finding the difficult vas

J. Cumming

It is not uncommon to be challenged by an impalpable vas in a male with a small scrotum, who is in a cold room.

My tip is to make a midline scrotal incision first and then palpate the spermatic cord with the thumb (or index finger) inside the incision. Start at the lower pole of the testis as far posterior as possible and sweep the pinched finger and thumb anteriorly until the vas is palpated (Fig. 46). At this point the vas and cord can be infiltrated with lignocaine and the vas mobilized in the preferred manner.

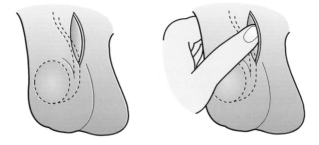

Figure 46

Tying the knot in a vasectomy made easier

D.J. Jones

For those people who still carry out vasectomies and continue to use an 'open' method this simple trick makes ligation of the looped-back vas a little easier. Once the vas has been dissected free and tented up, a pair of sharp mosquito artery forceps is inserted through the apex off the inverted U, sweeping the vessels downwards (a). Two mosquito forceps are then placed on the vas with the tips pointing downwards (b). A portion of the vas is excised (c) and the forceps are turned upwards producing a loop like a shepherd's crook (d). The now upturned mosquito makes ligation of the looped vas and removal of the mosquito much easier (e) (Fig. 47).

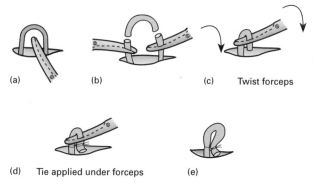

(a) (b) (c) Twist forceps

(d) Tie applied under forceps (e)

Figure 47

Vasectomy and preventing sperm granulomas

J. Cumming

If the ligature on the afferent (testicular) end of the vasectomy cuts through the vas or even falls off then a leak of sperms will create a sperm granuloma. To prevent this, double back the afferent end by applying two artery forceps, one at the free end and the other 1–2 cm proximally. Apply a ligature to the end and then take the ligature under the second artery forceps and tie the ligature again (Fig. 48). There should be a loop of vas as a result and hopefully less chance of sperm leak.

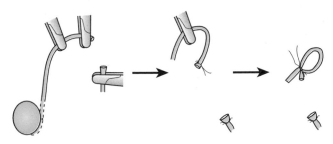

Figure 48

End-to-end vasovasostomy

J.C. Gingell

Reversal of a vasectomy can be made technically very straightforward if the upper segment is dilated with Bowman's lacrimal duct probes. The lumen of the upper end is always collapsed and in this way can be readily dilated to match the size of the lumen of the lower end. Four separate identical 6/0 prolene double-ended sutures with round-bodied needles (Ethicon 8712) are passed from 'inside out' through all layers at each quadrant and left untied (Fig. 49a). A folded abdominal pack on either side of the surgical field gives a white background so that the fine suture material can be more readily seen and the first suture on either side can be placed under the pack and the second on top. The sutures are then carefully tied, drawing the severed ends of the vas together. The ends of the two opposing sutures are left long and held in artery forceps to steady the anastomotic site allowing the insertion of intervening sutures of the same material (Fig. 49b). The anastomosis can be rotated to allow further suture placement around the whole circumference (Fig. 49c). Loupes for magnification are an advantage.

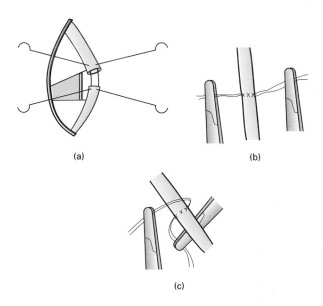

(a)

(b)

(c)

Figure 49

Easing the technical difficulty of microsurgical vasectomy reversal
M. Fox

The technique of microsurgical vasectomy reversal was ably described by Silber in 1977. Using 10/0 nylon and a two-layer interrupted end-to-end anastomosis (mucosa and then muscle wall), luminal patency can be achieved in virtually all cases, whether in the straight or convoluted part of the vas. The technique is not easy to master, and difficulty is often experienced because of disparity in the size of the proximal and distal lumina.

The method of anastomosis can be aided by a temporary insertion of a nylon splint which is removed before completion of the inner layer of sutures. A length of 3/0 nylon is introduced about 5 cm into the abdominal end of the vas and allowed to protrude from the lumen for some 2 cm. The ends of the vas are then brought into close contact and held steady in the approximating clamp. The nylon stent allows better visualization of the frequently narrower abdominal end of the vas and for correct and equidistant placing of the sutures. The protruding nylon end is used as a positioning handle in this respect (Fig. 50), enabling the lumen to be kept open until the last mucosal stitch has been inserted, after which time it is withdrawn before the last suture is tied.

Vasectomy reversal
Anonymous

The time lapse between the original vasectomy and its subsequent reversal is often long. It is now recognized that a proportion of men will, after time, develop testicular failure following vasectomy. This may be either as a result of the vasectomy itself or simply be due to aging.

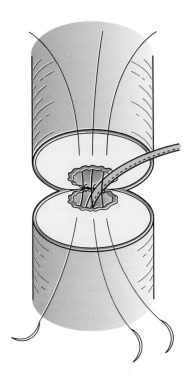

Figure 50

In such cases, there is an ideal opportunity to take a testicular biopsy to confirm the prescence of spermatogenesis at the time of undertaking the reversal. However, there is no need to wait for the result before proceeding with the reversal.

Where this tip can prove invaluable is in the post-operative period in that unhappy situation where no sperm appear in the ejaculate, and it may avert re-exploration of a 'technical failure' for what is not a technical problem but rather 'testicular failure'.

Making space for the undescended testicle
P.J. O'Boyle

When carrying out orchidopexy it is sometimes difficult to distend the scrotum sufficiently to make a suitable incision. This problem is easy to overcome by the use of a simple metal thimble which is easy to autoclave and sterilize. The thimble is introduced on the finger, distends the scrotum and allows an accurate skin incision to be made without difficulty.

Orchidopexy
J. Lawson

We have all been taught that the layers covering the spermatic cord represent reflections of those of the abdominal wall. In the mobilization of an inguinal undescended testis we all recognize the external spermatic fascia (external oblique) and the cremaster (internal oblique). How many of us, however, recognize the internal spermatic fascia — the thin, but remarkably strong, reflection of the transversalis fascia?

It may be the same operators that miss its extension — a 'mesentery' which attaches the vas and vessels to the posterior wall and extends forward between them. It is the failure to recognize this tube of internal spermatic fascia, and formally open it, which necessitates the subsequent dissection around the internal ring to divide the shredded transversalis reflection, eponymously known as Dennis Browne bands. Division of the extension between the vas and the vessels may give the cord that valuable extra 0.5 cm in length.

The hitch stitch for prevention of inguinoscrotal haematoma

P.J. O'Boyle

I have found this little tip, learned in Leeds, useful in preventing post-operative haematomas following inguinoscrotal or scrotal surgery such as inguinoscrotal hernias, large hydrocoeles or epididymal cysts. Under these circumstances conventional scrotal support and bandaging or drainage often prove ineffective. A hitch stitch using number 1 nylon tied over two dental rolls serves to hitch up the scrotal skin to the opposite abdominal wall (Fig. 51). This not only ablates the scrotal dead space, but also closes off the external inguinal ring, thereby preventing blood from tracking into the scrotal cavity. The hitch stitch is removed after 24 h.

Despite the appearance, patients tolerate this procedure remarkably well without increased pain or interference with micturition.

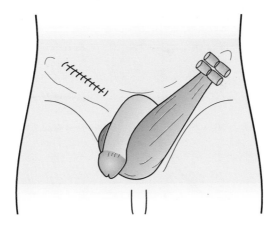

Figure 51

The unexpected bleed

Gaining control of vena caval haemorrhage using Foley catheters

P.J. O'Boyle

This manoeuvre, gleaned from Averil Mansfield, may prove life-saving following avulsion of the right renal vein or a tear in the inferior vena cava during a difficult radical nephrectomy. In such a case, the bleeding may be torrential and may prevent visualization and control of the defect.

A large abdominal pack is immediately placed over the

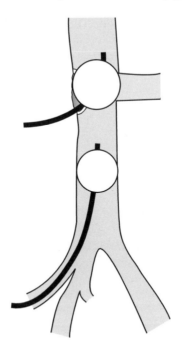

Figure 52

caval defect and pressure maintained by the assistant. A saphenofemoral cut down is made and a 10 F Foley catheter inserted via the saphenous vein to control proximal bleeding. A second 10 F Foley is then inserted through the rent and inflated at the point where the left renal vein enters the cava (Fig. 52). Control is thus achieved, allowing an occlusion clamp to be safely applied and the vein either repaired or patched. This manoeuvre dramatically reduces both caval blood loss and back bleeding from the opposite renal vein.

A different means of controlling caval haemorrhage using Foley catheters
J. Cumming

When in the above situation (see Gaining control of vena caval haemorrhage using Foley catheters, p. 112) it takes too long to expose the long saphenous vein if there is already a hole in the cava. In this case, insert two Foleys through the cavotomy, one up and one down, and sutures can be inserted around the catheters.

In such cases, it is worth remembering to clamp both Foleys or blood from the inferior vena cava pours down your underpants!

Unexpected surgical haemorrhage
R.W.M. Rees

On every general surgical tray sponge forceps are available and are usually used for preparing the patient. In the event of any unexpected massive haemorrhage any structure can be clamped with a sponge holder and the haemorrhage controlled, then the problem can be carefully identified and rectified. I have found this useful on occasions over the years. I do not claim originality as this advice was passed on to me by George Harrison of Derby.

Trauma to major veins
R.J. Luck

Place your finger over the tear or cut and suck out the wound dry. Your assistant then applies pressure with a 'swab on a stick' placed in each hand on either side of the cut or tear, allowing you to see and suture the defect (Fig. 53). In larger veins, e.g. the inferior vena cava, temporary control can be obtained in this way for long enough to place a partial occlusion vascular clamp across the injured vessel's wall.

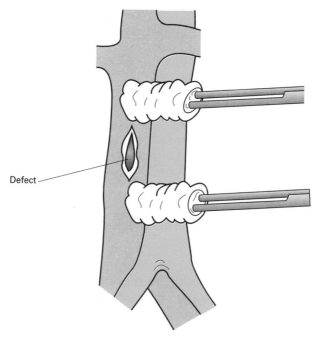

Defect

Figure 53

Index